# PRAISE

FOR

# CREATIVE MENOPAUSE

*Illuminating Women's Health & Spirituality*

**JOHN GRAY, Ph.D.**, author of *Men Are From Mars, Women Are From Venus*

"Creative Menopause expands the potential for the positive feminine experience, supports women to connect with their creative healing potential and inspires harmony in relationships."

**COUNTESS SALLY BALDWIN of Oxford, England**

"Farida Sharan combines thorough research with inspiring new ideas. Her work is not only informative, but also a joy to read"

**AHP PERSPECTIVE – Association for Humanistic Psychology**

The first forty–five pages are of great value for any woman, or for any person who may work with or live intimately with a menopausal woman. The depth and breadth of the experience is grasped eloquently here. All and all it is a shining example of the loving care a small press can bring to book design. I would recommend this as a gift to oneself or a loved woman of these years."

**ALTERNATIVE & COMPLEMENTARY THERAPIES JOURNAL (NY)**

"This book awakens a deeper appreciation for the currents of spirituality flowing through and influencing the cycles of the feminine experience."

**ROSEMARY GLADSTAR – Author *Herbal Healing for Women*, Sage Herbal School**

"Written from the heart, *Creative Menopause* is a beautifully inspirational and unique contribution to the growing body of literature exploring this stage of a woman's life. Farida takes us deep into the heart of the issues surrounding menopause, embracing the physical, spiritual and transformational processes that are occurring in our bodies and leads us ever so gently through the confusion to a place of self empowerment."

**NAPRA REVIEW – Spring 1995**

"Among the many books about menopause available today, this one stands out as taking an unusually holistic – and refreshing – approach. There are the expected chapters covering the physical symptoms and treatment of menopause, but the book focuses primarily on the emotional changes that occur during this passage and on what is ultimately a spiritual transition. Written with authenticity and sensitivity, this is a freeing and empowering work that will be welcomed by many women."

**DAN POYNTER – Para Publishing**

"A much needed book, very nicely done. Congratulations."

**PENELOPE YOUNG ANDRADE – L.C.S.W., San Diego**

" I bow to your courage, your clarity and your light."

### JOHN CHITTY– President of the American Polarity Association

"This book combines practicality and inspiration in a wonderfully eloquent way. It will be valuable for so many. Women obviously are the primary beneficiaries of the information which will help them understand and find positive solutions to the challenges of the many mental, emotional and physical events associated with menopause. But it will also be extremely valuable to men, who will gain deep insight into the experience, and to caregivers of both genders and all ages and disciplines.

The practical side of the book is its clear and comprehensive descriptions of the many sides of menopause and the many holistic strategies available to the seeker of natural answers to feminine health problems. Farida ia also very practical in her explanation of the many solid reasons for avoiding the drugs–and–surgery approach of conventional health care. Before this book, this information has not been widely available in such a concise and focused form.

This is a call for liberation: freedom from the pain of various aspects of the situation of course, but also freedom in a much larger sense. By encouraging personal responsibility, self–understanding and spiritual awareness as integral parts of the healing process, Farida speaks to the deepest dimensions of the quest for health and balance shared by all humanity."

### DR. ANTHEA GUINESS

"The writing is beautiful – nice flow, vivid descriptions. The silence of our mothers, our mothers' mothers, and *their* mothers, is amazing! All this information should have been part of a tradition they added to and passed on. Your book is a legacy I didn't know existed."

### MICHAEL TIERRA – Author of *Way of Herbs*

"Written with compassion and authority, *Creative Menopause* is a gift from one of the leaders of the herbal renaissance. It should help to guide the many goddess women whose dedication to gaia and nature makes them worthy of empowerment as they enter the threshold of their wisdom years."

### SHARON PORTER – Co-Founder of the Polarity Institute and Registered Polarity Practitioner

"Your book is wonderful! It's really a whole woman work, pulling together the practical and empowering information we women need to transform ourselves and our world. My clients can't wait to get their hands on *Creative Menopause* and share it with their friends and daughters. It's empowering at every level while compiling practical information and treatments that women can and will use. It also comes from the gut of a woman who walks her talk. Revolutionary! Evolutionary!

It has helped me feel better about taking the time for rest and repose which my body sometimes yearns for but which does not fit societal expectations. I'm also feeling at peace with having more fat on my body than I used to, appreciating my goddess shape as important for natural, post–menopausal estrogen production."

### CONSCIOUS LIVING MAGAZINE – Australia

"Aptly sub–titled '*Illuminating Women's Health & Spirituality*' the author strongly advocates that women in their 30's reclaim the responsibility for the care of their own health in order to take themselves through menopause in the most healthy way."

### RED ROSE

"Realize Your Spiritual Potential. This is a beautifully written and illustrated inspirational book. It is a must read for women wanting empowering information about this important and sacred mid-life transition. Highly recommended for both its practical and spiritual content."

# Illuminating Women's Health & Spirituality

# Creative Menopause

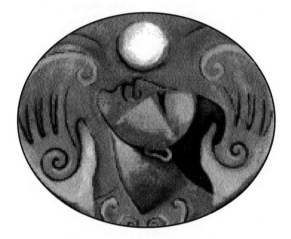

# Illuminating Women's Health & Spirituality

# Creative Menopause

## Farida Sharan MDMA ND MH

**Wisdome Press**
A Division of School of Natural Medicine
Boulder, Colorado

WISDOME PRESS
School of Natural Medicine
Post Office Box 7369
Boulder, Colorado 80306–7369, USA
TEL: (888) 593–6173
FAX: (888) 593–6733
www.purehealth.com

10 9 8 7 6 5 4 3

The author or the publisher are not responsible for your health, your disease or your healing journey. We do not
accept any responsibility for problems, adverse reactions or consequences resulting from the use of any remedy,
suggestion, guidance, procedure or preparation included in *Creative Menopause – Illuminating Women's Health &
Spirituality*. We recommend you consult a qualified professional health care provider. We wish you joy of healing
on your journey.

Library of Congress Catalog Card Number: 94–76389


Sharan, Farida
    Creative Menopause: illuminating women's health and
spirituality / Farida Sharan.
    p. cm.
    Includes index.
    ISBN 1-57093-002-3
1. Menopause  2. Menopause–Psychological Aspects.  3. Women – Health and hygiene.  4. Naturopathy.
5. Mind and body.  6. Menopause – Nutritional aspects.  7. Herbs – Therapeutic use.  8. Self Actualization
(Psychology).    I. Title

RG186.S53 1994                    618.1'75
                                 QBI94–779

Printed and bound on acid free paper in Boulder, Colorado, United States of America.

*This book is dedicated to the sacred feminine –*

*all souls are feminine before the divine.*

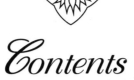

# Contents

# Acknowledgments

This book has been an amazing creative adventure. I have received so much loving support during its creation that first I must thank this wondrous universe for showering me with its abundance – and an abun–dance it was – this adventure into writing and self publishing.

First I thank Michelle Steyskal, my capable assistant, for helping me paste–up the first edition. The school office was full of lotuses, inspirational art, paste, paper, music and laughter and we prepared the master copies to reach Australia before my lectures and workshops. I began to work on the book again after my return in December and during this phase I give my deepest appreciation to my editor, David Joel, for his thoughtful and patient suggestions, as he helped me organize and weave my ideas into a clear and consistent flow.

The search for a cover concept manifested dramatically when I remembered a beautiful artcard I had bought on the island of Kauai in Hawaii. On impulse I wrote to the artist, Mara Friedman, and received a bountiful envelope of exquisite and inspiring art, along with permission to use her images. Sandra Patterson–Slaydon's careful editing brought many important considerations to my attention. Phone calls and letters from friends and colleagues – Shady Sirotkin, Dr. Anthea Margi Becker of Mussoorie in the Himalayas in India, Elspeth Taimre of Western Australia, Dr. Jesse Hanley of Malibu in California, Katrama Brooks of Kauai in Hawaii, my sister Thais Baker of Vancouver in Canada and my daughters Casel and Chalice Melendy – all offered important suggestions. John Chitty, President of the American Polarity Therapy Association gave valued advice and support during the last stages of editing and design, as did Sharon Porter, the co-founder of the Polarity Institute. Incredible creative sessions with Lisa Hertzi and Julie Noyes Long brought the front and back covers to life. My dear soul sister, Tamara Matthews, contributed suggestions regarding the explanations of emotional concepts. Brian Vanduzee gave invaluable advice to help bring together the medical section. Thank you.

All through this whirlwind of effort, synchronicity and grace, Carolyn Oakley supported the project with her capable computer skills, devoting weekend and evening time with a warm heart, a great sense of fun and good humor. Shawn Collins offered generous computer support and advice whenever we had a problem – many thanks! Proofreader Richard Haight helped to polish and refine the final draft. David Joel put together the index with graceful synchronicity. Meanwhile, Tara Goldfarb–Elias, the School of Natural Medicine office manager, kept the administration going with enthusiasm, providing a background for this creative venture.

Above and beyond all, I thank my beloved spiritual master for the continuous grace and mercy which He showers on my life. Without His love which flows and flowers in everything I do, nothing could be accomplished. Everything is offered in His service.

# ILLUSTRATORS

**Mara Friedman's** inspiring original paintings grace our cover and are placed throughout the text. Her images focus upon and reflect the deep Feminine nature. She explores the many aspects of Woman and gives form to Her fluid cycles of awareness. Mara's women, whether in action, repose, prayer or in dreams, symbolize the unifying connection between the outer world of nature and the inner world of the soul. The goddess and angelic archetypal images complement the intent of this book to support women to prepare for, identify with, and experience their divinity. Mara was born in California in 1955 and shares her time between the island of Kauai in Hawaii and the Oregon countryside. To inquire about paintings, prints and artcards:

P.O. Box 23, Lorane, Oregon 97451, U.S.A. (800) 701–6984
email: mara@newmoonvisions.com   website: www.newmoonvisions.com

**Sandra Patterson–Slaydon's** exquisite watercolor, *Farida's Dream*, the cover of *Herbs of Grace*, is also featured in the Diamond Menopause section. It is a visionary painting from her essence, created in alignment with my work on both *Herbs of Grace* and *Creative Menopause – Illuminating Women's Health & Spirituality*. Sandra is my dear soul sister and resonates with the deepest purpose of this offering to women.

**Peter Torensma's** visionary painting *The Elemental Eye* is placed in both the Elemental Emotions Brow and Crown Spiritual Centers pages. Beautiful art cards of his paintings are available from Aurora Productions, Pb 8174, 1802 KD Alkmaar – Holland.

# Illustrations

# Movements of the Soul

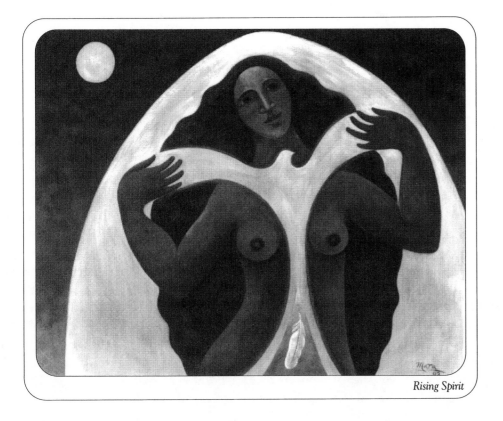

*Rising Spirit*

Movements of the soul begin during conception when the divine spirit merges with the microcosmic physical. The journey continues in utero as the soul gathers layers of astral, mental and physical bodies around its essence. Emergence into the world at birth marks another transition, and continuing growth measures the journey of the soul. During life we move through continuous change, recognizing and celebrating from time to time the transition from one cycle to another. The girl child emerges into the maiden and the maiden into the lover, the wife and the mother. Each movement signifies the departure from the ending cycle as well as the entrance into the new. At the entrance to each new cycle we are honored, often celebrating the change with a birthday party, a wedding, a birthing or christening ceremony until we reach mid–life and menopause. Then the celebration stops and the silence and shame begins. This is where women go underground into darkness, disease and denial. Instead of honoring this growth cycle as it continues into the spiritual realms of being, menopause is regarded as a disease and a disturbance. It seems as though our world admires only the physical growing and ripening. Once the physical fullness begins to decline and the soul begins its movement out of this world, we do not know how to value and respect the wisdom and the more invisible emerging spiritual potential.

Mid–life is a transition, a time of change, a time of completion and a time of beginning. It is an opportunity to discover the vast reservoir of resources gathered during our lives and make them available for personal evolutionary processes. It is also a creative challenge because at this time, perhaps more than any other, women have the opportunity to transform negativity into positivity and darkness into light. We take what is essentially an ending and create a beginning, a self–birth that flows from the very essence of our being.

When we take up the challenge of a creative and spiritual mid–life we can turn this fertile opportunity into our crowning glory. We can create a flowering and fruitful transition that is more exciting than building a million–dollar company, deep–sea diving or trekking in the Himalayas. There is no greater frontier than exploring our inner world and bringing forth meaning and purpose into our lives. The change of life gives every woman the opportunity to transform the straw of possibility into the gold of creativity, to emerge enriched and strengthened, fully born into the wise woman and the elder who joyfully celebrates the inner child and contains all aspects of the feminine. It also gives us the opportunity to share this deeper level of our creative essence with our family, friends and community.

After setting the stage with the Movements of the Soul introduction, we look at The Mid–Life Threshold. This section is followed by My Creative Change and Life Cycles of the Feminine. Then we turn the kaleidoscope of our vision to Diamond Menopause to awaken our perception to the different facets and thresholds of experience that call for our attention and demand recognition and integration during menopause. After presenting Physical Healing – Spinning Straw Into Gold we move on to Emotional Clearing – Weeding the Garden of Life, Cosmic Sexuality – Lifting Up The Power, Mental Winnowing – Separating Myths From Truths, Spiritual Transformation – Dissolving into the Divine, Medical Realities – Facing the Dragons, and The Honored Elder. These sections are followed by the glossary, index and appendices.

The extensive Physical Healing section is divided into three. After presenting the processes we learn to work with during our change, purification, regeneration and transformation, the second section describes how our organs, glands and body systems are related to the mid–life change of life. Menopause can easily become confused with symptoms caused by the development of individual aging processes and chronic conditions. Therefore, it is important to understand that many of the bitter seeds that flower in disease and discomfort during menopause were sown in earlier years by stress, repressed or excessive mental attitudes and emotions, and disordered digestion, in the soil of our body, emotions, mind, spirit and life. Above all we learn that mid–life is a individual process, with many different influences and factors to consider.

The third section of Physical Healing looks at the different symptoms and conditions that develop during aging and menopause and the ways that our period cycles and hormones change. For each health condition we learn how to support, balance and heal uncomfortable symptoms using herbs, homeopathy, diet, supplements, flower essences and natural treatments, as well as how to explore emotional, mental and spiritual causes of physical symptoms. We also learn how to prevent the development of aging and menopausal problems, by knowing which organs, glands and body systems need to be cared for during the earlier life cycles of the feminine and which ones need to be strengthened and supported during our mid–life transition.

In Emotional Clearing – Weeding the Garden of Life, we introduce Carl Jung's individuation process and the integration of the shadow. We then explore emotional clearing through the lens of the Elements of Life. We discover that we can make the most of the opportunity that mid–life offers by challenging our unborn selves to release our negativity, our shadow, our self destructiveness, our unconsciousness and our fear. We also learn how to transform our emotional passions, so that we can utilize their energies as gifts to support our personal evolution.

This is a book written from my heart, soul and experience. I have not included information on synthetic hormones or medical treatments which are not part of my experience. If you wish information on these other realities please read the works of experts in these areas. Above all, explore, research and be true to your self. Find your path of truth.

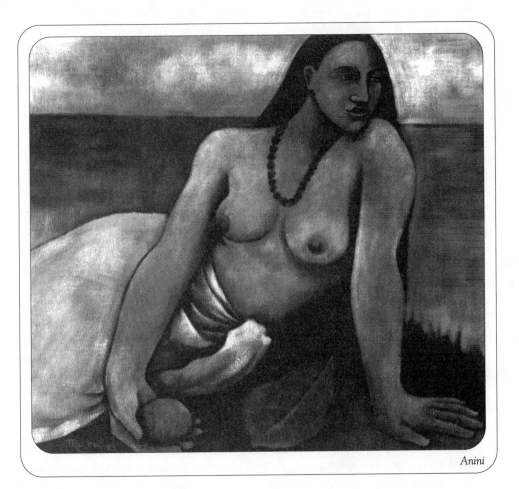

*Anini*

Mid–life is a time to clear the weeds that have grown from our fears, our carelessness, our ignorance and our negativity. It is an opportunity to release that which has stolen our creative, joyful and spiritual energies. It is a time to make our life a garden of beauty, displaying the flowers, fruits and seeds of our love. It is a time to become who we really are, who we always wanted to be and who we always knew we were. It is a time for joy, for celebration and for service. It is a time of harvest, of clearing and gathering our energy for a deeper inner life. It is a time to become timeless. It is a time of richness beyond imagination, a preparation for an even greater journey, the return of our soul to its source, our soul journey home.

Cosmic Sexuality – Lifting Up The Power considers all the influences we have received during our lives that have formed our sexuality in its many facets, dimensions and realities. This helps us clear the way for a fresh beginning that flows from our deepest essence and our truth.

Mental Winnowing – Separating Myths and Truths reflects the ancient process of separating grain from chaff. We examine both the myths and truths of aging, sexuality, mental abilities, family, society, work, medicine, creativity and spirituality. We find that once we have freed aging and menopause from cultural, community and family conditioning, we can look with fresh eyes on what mid–life really is, a creative opportunity that moves us through a transition to the rich years of wisdom and the inner life. We learn to seek role models for guidance and inspiration. We learn we must separate menopause from our negative attitudes, from cultural expectations, from advertising messages and from our own constitutional aging process.

The Spiritual Transformation – Dissolving into the Divine section points the way to truth, the future, and our ultimate divine reality.

Medical Realities – Facing the Dragons offers a fresh look at the current medical system. Now that we have expanded our vision to include many other possibilities and approaches to aging, mid–life and menopause, we can work with and use the positive aspects of modern medicine to support our menopausal process. We can also learn how to question and explore the options and suggestions and determine which medical treatments are beneficial for our condition. This prepares us for our role as The Honored Elder.

We conclude with a glossary, appendices on herbs and supplements to use before, during and after menopause, index and information on books, videos, tapes, resources, study programs and ordering information.

This book is recommended to be used together with Farida Sharan's book *Herbs of Grace – Becoming Independently Healthy* which contains specific, detailed information and instructions on the use of herbal instructions, herbal formulae, nourishment through healing diets, and herbal and naturopathy treatments. Although I have presented as much information as possible within this book, the use of herbs and  natural treatments is a life study requiring personal guidance from professionals, gradual learning through personal experience, as well as study and reference from excellent books. There are classes, seminars, correspondence courses, school, conferences and symposiums available in most parts of the country, where a wealth of herbal knowledge can be gained. I would encourage everyone to learn as much as possible about natural medicine. *Herbs of Grace* also contains the story of the my healing from breast cancer, the source of wisdom and  experience that is the foundation of my approach to health and healing.

# The Mid-Life Threshold

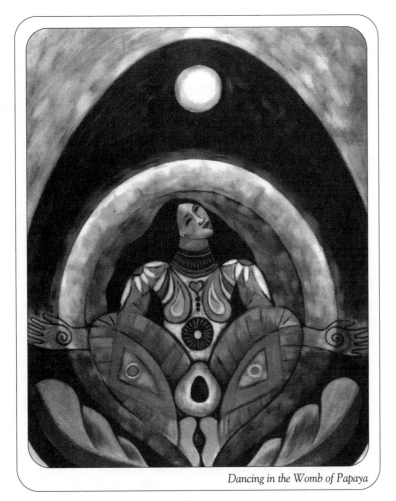

*Dancing in the Womb of Papaya*

Mid–life is a doorway, a threshold, an initiation, a transition and a unique experience for every woman. The orthodox medical system regards aging and menopause as illnesses and recognizes them as markets for financial gain. Other cultures celebrate menopause and see it as a transition that leads to the spiritual life and our years as a wise woman, grandmother and elder. Let us examine the realities and the possibilities that define aging and menopause and realize that now, at this time, more than any other, women have the opportunity and the challenge to create a personal experience that is both an adventure and a victory. We are on the leading edge of a time when we are redefining feminine roles and feminine experience. We are presently breaking fertile ground for generations of women to come. We are opening the way for the expression of the feminine essence in this world, making what has been invisible, visible. Each woman's contribution is significant and valuable.

Menopause begins toward the end of our fertility cycle when our hormones set in motion the changes which lead to the cessation of periodic bleeding. Menopause is more than a pause of our monthly cycle. It is a transition that takes place on many different levels. It is the end of our fertility cycle and the beginning of cosmic fertility – our life beyond the cycles of the moon, the tides of the ocean, and the rise and fall of blood in our womb. This may happen before the age of forty, or during the forties and fifties. For some women it happens quickly, either instantly after surgery, or just naturally. For others it is a process that takes many years. Women experience individual reactions, emotions, symptoms and conditions in varying degrees. Hormones also trigger the release of repressed, denied and unfinished experiences and energies in physical, emotional, sexual, mental and spiritual aspects of our lives. On one level the question of what menopause truly is needs to be separated from aging, chronic disease, emotional disorders and the effects of stressful and negligent lifestyles. On another level, because menopause comes when we are reaping the harvest of our past actions, these personal realities form the background of our transition, making each menopause experience completely unique.

Menopause is set into motion when the ovaries slow down estrogen production. The follicular stimulating hormones (FSH) continue to increase as they attempt to stimulate the ovaries to prepare egg cells, disturbing the hypothalamus gland, which controls blood temperature, sleep and energy. The autonomic nervous system, which normally regulates the unconscious functions of breathing, digestion, blood pressure and heartbeats, is also affected, causing disturbances and producing uncomfortable symptoms.

Hormones continue to be produced during and after menopause, at lowered though consistent levels, in the ovaries, body fat and adrenals. The ovaries also produce androgens, which are hormones (similar to male hormones) that promote muscle strength, vaginal elasticity and sex drive, and play an important part in general health. Androgens are converted into estrogen in direct relation to the amount of peripheral body fat. Menopausal women are naturally more full–bodied in response to this need. Women who strive for the lean look of youth are short–changing themselves more than they realize because they minimize estrogen production due to lack of body fat. However, excessive body weight is also to be avoided, as it increases the risk of heart, breast, uterine and digestive diseases.

Healthy women can produce enough androgen–based estrogen to protect themselves from uncomfortable menopausal body changes, but not all women are able to generate sufficient amounts. The ovaries of healthy women do not shrivel and cease functioning. They continue to produce androgens after menopause and never stop producing them for the rest of women's lives. How can we maintain a healthy level of natural hormones? How can we prepare for menopause? How can we preserve the function of our body systems, glands and organs that affect our menopause and our life after the change? Women can overcome personal health problems by utilizing the opportunity mid-life offers to transform darkness into light, negativity into positivity, and imbalance into dynamic equilibrium.

When women become menopausal, all that we have pushed down, denied and left unfinished rises to the surface to be cleared, so that we have the opportunity to become wise, fulfilled, and reach our highest potential as elders and grandmothers. During this change, emotions are powerful. Blocked energy rises. Traumas demand to be released. If we do not flow with the change and transform and release negative energy, illness manifests. Life situations we have endured now become intolerable. Change is inevitable. Cooperation with the creative menopause allows us to cut through our bitter harvest, pull out weeds, prune rampant growth, enjoy the fruits and flowers of the garden of our lives, and sow potent seeds for the future.

Reproductive diseases develop over a long period of time and contain many causes and influences in their creation. Generally overlooked by the medical profession, however, are the causes related to negative emotions and mental attitudes. The tensions and changes in body chemistry produced by these repressed negative energies can create an imploding self–destructive climate that manifests in symptoms according to individual weaknesses and constitution. Through internalizing unresolved emotional pain, women unconsciously injure their reproductive organs and develop cancer, cysts, fibroids and reproductive diseases and other symptoms and conditions. Diet, stress and lifestyle, together with hereditary weaknesses, also play their part in creating disease. Healing requires women to soften, feel their pain and plunge deeply through feeling to their ground of truth, which reflects spirituality and compassion. It also requires discipline to change life habits, time and energy to turn the tide of self–destructive processes, courage to look at the truth, and love to allow receptivity to healing.

As women, we spend a total of four years during an average life span releasing our monthly flow of blood. Have we experienced the shame or the nuisance of blood, or have we celebrated the gold of blood? Have we enjoyed our monthly cycle and mourned its loss, or have we despised it and can't wait to have it end? What attitudes and emotions have we constellated around our monthly cycle? As our cycles change during menopause we have the opportunity to clear negative patterns and to free ourselves for healing and integration. Menopause can be the most important stage of our lives if we use it as an opportunity to jettison all that is unnecessary and learn to live from simplicity, truth, clarity and purpose.

It has been documented that women who have not had periods for many years begin them again when they fall in love. Love affects hormones. Divine love, spirituality, unconditional love and joyful service, enable love, health, hormones, and energy to flow. Let's make our menopause conscious and always be in love. Love does not have to be just for a specific man or woman, or only for our own children. Love can be for all of humanity and all of life. Love can be a constant state of bliss from which we live our lives.

Yes, grieve your losses. Yes, release your fears. Yes, let go of your desires. Live and practice a spiritual path that leads to peace and contentment. Live life fully and joyfully so that each moment becomes an opportunity for deeper self–understanding and self–transformation. Focus the diamond of attention on the eternal, not on what is passing away. Walk toward the end of life as if it were the beginning. Walk toward death as if you were walking toward birth. Walk toward darkness as if you were walking toward light.

# MENOPAUSE IS...

*an opportunity*

*an individual process*

*the end of physical fertility and the monthly flow of blood*

*a process that lasts several years*

*the opening of cosmic fertility*

*emotional, mental and spiritual, as well as physical*

*a celebration*

*a letting go*

*a time for integration*

*a time to make changes*

*a time for dealing with unfinished business*

*a time to stop holding down pain, shame and fear*

*a time to dig down and dive deep into your interior being*

*a time to seek, to reach, to fly – to soar higher and higher*

*a time to be outrageously yourself*

*a time to speak your truth*

*a time to give energy to your spiritual life*

*a time for healing*

*a time of preparation for the rest of your life*

# MENOPAUSE IS NOT...

*a chronic disease*

*just in your mind*

*an unspeakable shame*

*something to be afraid of*

*the end of your creativity*

*something to ignore and deny*

# DOES NOT...

*diminish your sexuality*

*make you worthless*

*make you old*

*dry you up*

# POSITIVE ROLE MODELS

*Saint*

*Wise Woman*

*Star of your own life*

*Medicine woman, healer*

*Goddess*

*Crone*

*Wife*

*Recluse*

*Adventurer*

*Career woman*

*Muse that inspires creativity*

*Artist, writer, musician, dancer, teacher*

*Social, charitable, ecological or political activist*

*Happy menopausal woman who loves being herself*

*Mother, God Mother, Grand Mother, Great Grand Mother*

How do you see yourself as a mid–life woman? What positive or negative role models did you have when you were growing up? Was there an older woman who inspired you to become like her? Was there a complete absence of positive role models? Did you fear that you might end up like one of the negative role models in your young life? Remember your mother, godmother, grandmother, aunt, teacher, movie star, or any other older woman who might have been in your life. Let yourself receive the gift of their positivity, and release the rest, so that you can become yourself. Do not act out or continue their limitations. Make your dreams come true. Set an example for future generations. Do not feel deprived if there is no one, because that gives you the opportunity to create an authentic life.

# My Creative Change

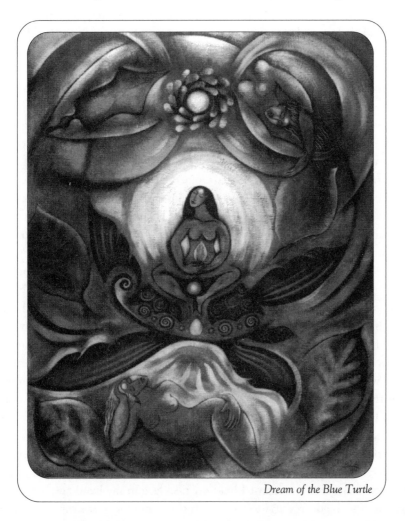

*Dream of the Blue Turtle*

I had no concept of menopause when I was a young woman. During my training it was glossed over. None of the women in my life even talked about it. Then, at thirty–five years of age I began my work as a Doctor of Natural Medicine in a London gynecological practice and in my own practice in Cambridge, England. I received direct referrals from my colleagues who were medical doctors, from the Bristol Cancer Clinic and from other allopathic and complementary practitioners and doctors. Menopausal women became my patients.

During consultations older women talked about their change, but every woman explained it in a different way. Some would talk about similar symptoms, like hot flashes, but their experiences would be different. I soon realized there was no way to treat menopause itself, and began to work completely individually with each woman. I used iris analysis to gain an understanding of the inner ecology of their body organs, systems and glands, their constitutional strengths and weaknesses, the effectiveness of their eliminative organs and levels of toxicity or inflammation. This analysis, together with an in–depth consultation exploring their history, use of medical drugs or surgeries, diet, stress levels, emotions, mental attitudes, and work and lifestyle irregularities, guided their individual treatment program. Over the years this developed into a comprehensive system of natural medicine based on therapeutic dietary, herbal and naturopathic purification and rejuvenation that consistently gave results. Many of the cases were documented by medical tests both before and after treatment. One medical doctor I worked with said she never knew that such tissue changes were possible. It was evident the system produced profound healing results when women dedicated themselves to following their treatment programs.

A common thread began to appear in each case I worked with. I began to see that each woman had woven herself and her life into a knot that had become too tangled to undo. During my consultations I searched for a way to help women free themselves. I saw my clients regularly so they had the opportunity to talk about their problems and begin the process of change and letting go. This approach eventually developed into the complete healing system of purification, regeneration and transformation outlined in *Herbs of Grace*. This process combines herbal formulae created individually for each client, together with dietary changes, Bach flower remedies, home naturopathy treatments, and referrals for massage, reflexology, polarity therapy, chiropractic, osteopathy, homeopathy, and psychotherapy whenever necessary. The results spoke for themselves and many women who healed their illnesses went on to study with the School of Natural Medicine and become natural health practitioners and educators themselves.

After having treated hundreds of menopausal women, my menopause became a reality for me at forty–two years of age. I still remember the day quite clearly. I was in consultation at the London clinic with one of the female leaders of the Brahma Kumaris spiritual group, an Indian woman from the head temple in the northern deserts of India. During our consultation I suddenly felt a burning wave rise from my depths and spread throughout my body and then over my face. My neck burned red hot. For a moment I could hardly breathe. Without revealing any discomfort, I continued the consultation. The woman and her two female companions seemed unaware of any change in me. My skin prickled from the heat. No sooner did one wave reside then another one came. For a moment I held my necklace in my hand and it nearly burned my hand. I began to breathe deeply and to work with this inner process. I was also very involved in my work with my client, so I proceeded with the consultation, although it seemed as if another level of my being had opened up below the one that was functioning professionally on the surface. For an hour I was like two people, one performing her work and another deeply involved with waves of heat and energy that were creating a reservoir of completely new experiences within my being.

That night after I left the clinic I kept to my regular schedule. After visiting the Turkish baths I took my usual walk through London. Instead of walking for a mile or two and then having dinner, I kept walking and walking. It seemed as though I could not get enough of walking. The heat waves started again and the cool misty winter air refreshed me. I had an abundance of energy, and was neither hungry nor tired. Now that I did not have to talk or work,

I gave myself totally to the experience. I walked without fear through dark London streets and down by the Thames. I walked for hours into the night and did not tire. Finally about midnight I reached the University Women's Club where I lodged when I worked in London. Once I settled myself into my room and was able to completely focus on my interior life, I realized that I felt huge and vast within myself, as though the person that I always thought of as me was just a small part of a greater me. I remember saying to myself, "I feel like the Grand Canyon. I'm just layers and layers. This is Grand Canyon consciousness."

Perhaps because I had healed my own cancer and spent nearly twenty years purifying and regenerating my body and living a simple healthy lifestyle, developing an intimate dialogue with the different aspects of my being, I was able to welcome, explore and enjoy these hot flashes. Perhaps because I had meditated for years I was able to be sensitive to these inner energies. Perhaps because I had taken treatments of acupuncture, rolfing, Alexander technique and other therapies, I was open to receive these changes. Whatever the reason, I did not resist them. I did not even dwell on whether they were uncomfortable. I was totally fascinated with the movement of heat and energy and this opening up of a vast dimension of my being that I never knew existed before. The hot flashes went beyond the physical. My experience opened deep layers of primal emotion and ancient memory which were illuminated and infused with spirituality, truth and powerful energy.

This aspect of my menopausal process continued for about six months. The flashes became a part of my life. I looked forward more and more to my time in London each week where the great long night walks seemed the perfect time for integration. Sometimes when a particular flash would illuminate a part of my being, filling me with spiritual love and longing, I would stop on a street or a corner and just stand, transfixed with the beauty of the energy. People would walk by and around me and sometimes I noticed their glances, but I was not concerned. I was in a state of ecstasy, accessing profound levels of love and longing within my being.

However, the flashes also began to bring up painful memories, emotions and increased sexual desire. It was as though my entire being was flaming, clearing, increasing, purifying and transforming. As overpowering as this experience was, I concealed it completely. I told no one. At that time it was pure experience and I could not have written or talked about it as I do now. My staff knew that I was going through something unusual, but true to the English custom, no one asked any questions. It was amazing that no matter how intense the experience was, how difficult the release from my depths, or how powerful the emotion, I never stopped functioning on the surface of my life. I carried a great and marvelous and exciting secret, and I felt strong and radiant, but it was not connected to anything or anyone outside of me. I was in love with my self, my greater self, my higher self, with the divine within my own being, that was helping me, teaching me, making me expand and grow, and it was wonderful. Even when the releases were difficult they were surrounded and supported by love and an intense electric energy that sustained me through the process.

Toward the fourth month the releases increased in purity, beauty and intensity. As I grounded more deeply in my being, I began to perceive the reality of my life around me in a different way. My martyr persona was dissolving. I could no longer do things the way that I always had. I saw more deeply. It was as though I read people's minds and motives and feelings. I looked at my life and realized I would have to change.

These realizations awakened a new cycle of my menopausal experience, and deeper levels of mental and emotional pain surfaced. Absolute truth was building up and I did not have the language to speak, and did not know how to untie the tangled knot of my life. I saw that I was all things. I saw that everything that I always thought was not me was there inside. I saw that I could be anything, from the very worst to the very highest. I also saw that my life had unfolded exactly as it was meant, and now I understood from pure experience the deeper meaning of words like destiny and karma.

This deeper level of realization caused emotional pain which became mingled with the ecstasy. It was not enough to just experience the pure energy, it also had a purpose. It now became clear that I would have to change my life. The pain came because the raw truth revealing itself before me demanded change, but I could not imagine how to accomplish the change. I meditated until it seemed as if my light of consciousness was the only beacon in a great sea of internal and external darkness. I saw that my present life was intolerable, but I had no new direction or path. I no longer was able to exist in the ivory tower of my fantasy. This new level of truth and awareness demanded integration into my life. I knew I would have to break free from my old life, but I didn't know how.

While all of these truths, realities and emotions were surfacing from my inner life, my outer life was also demanding resolution. In my profession I was being slandered publicly by the owners of a rival school who went to great lengths, expense and energy to try to destroy my reputation and my work. In my private life, my children were angry with me because they wanted me to leave England and my husband and return to America. Even though I now wanted to do this, I did not know how it could be accomplished. My husband and I lived in opposite ends of the same large house and had separate lives. I was not yet prepared to make these changes and the pressure collected, like before an earthquake or a volcanic eruption. This was supremely uncomfortable, but I realize now that it was a necessary stage of the transformation process.

A friend suggested I have a consultation with Liz Green, a respected English Jungian analyst who was also an author and an astrologer. I had reached the point where I needed to talk to an expert. I felt I was losing myself to such a degree in this formless descent that I was going to go mad. But I was able to hold myself together, until at last I walked into her consulting room.

She looked at me and even before I sat down, she said, "Are you going through this on your own or are you getting help?"

I looked at her, startled, and replied, "On my own."

"You are very fortunate to be able to have this pure experience of the descent and the shadow. This is the best way if you are strong enough. Most people need to talk it through and have support, but that waters it down, while others have breakdowns or go mad. You are fortunate to be able to endure the pure experience."

She knew exactly from my birth data the depth and intensity of the experience that I was going through. I walked out of her office with a fresh perception. She had provided me with exactly what I needed to continue the inner work on my own. She had told me about the integration of the shadow and the individuation process. Now I knew that other people had gone through this descent, and had not only survived, but emerged victorious. Now I knew it was a recognized and documented process. Just knowing this eased the pressure. I was able to surrender and allow transformation to take place without fear or resistance.

Soon after, when I was walking one night in the central London theater district, I turned up Shaftesbury Avenue and saw the Silver Moon bookstore. I stopped for a moment to look in the window and saw a book with the title *Descent to the Goddess* by Sylvia Pereira. On the cover was an illustration of an ancient sculpture of a woman with large hips and thighs. I was transfixed. That image was exactly how my body had changed during this experience. I had taken on that shape. I had not been able to understand why I was gaining weight although I was walking more than I ever had and eating less. First thing next morning I returned to purchase the book and to browse and buy others. Thus began my study of psychology, the archetypes, the goddess myths and the works of New Age and feminist pioneers who were striving to bring this uncharted arena of human experience into print.

I had not read for several years and now I could not stop reading. I absorbed the books on a very deep level. Their truths went into my being and became part of me. I understood everything because I had experienced it. I was on fire with a passion to explore and discover this whole new realm of life. Soon my consulting and teaching expanded. I was able to perceive deeper currents in the lives of the patients who came to see me about their health problems, and I shared this new wisdom with my students. I prepared and gave lectures on my experience of the integration of the shadow, and how repressed or excessive emotions created feminine reproductive diseases. A deeper layer of truth had opened in my life.

It seemed as if I were expanding and contracting simultaneously, and although the process was intense, even uncomfortable, it was also incredibly rich and exciting. The increase of inspired creativity from my essence was matched by the closing down of all that I had been before. This was painful for me because I could see no way out of my situation or how to make the necessary changes. My life had become too complicated. I wondered what would happen. I was teetering on the wall of conflict, afraid to move, seeing only potential disaster in every direction. The only thing I could do was get up every day and do the best I could in every area of my life, living the transition and the mystery, and waiting to see how and when change would manifest.

I felt committed to my marriage because of my spiritual path. I managed a large school and felt a deep level of responsibility for my staff, students and patients. I could not imagine how I would find time to find a place to move to and go through a divorce. There were so many responsibilities with my three children, I could not risk loss of income. My life situation seemed unchangeable. Although I still performed at optimum levels in my professional life, the moment my daily responsibilities were over, I was plunged into despair. The only antidote was to connect with the divine through meditation, and every day I gave thanks that this great gift was in my life. Slowly a dull, flat, unfeeling depression seeped into every aspect of my being. Gone was my natural love and enthusiasm and optimism for daily life. Although I seemed empty, unnourished, exhausted and unable to move or change, somehow every day I was able to take care of my home, my family and my work. When I look back on this period it seems a miracle that I was supported internally as I went through this amazing inner and outer transformation. My spiritual path was clearly my source of inner strength and inspiration.

Over the years I have learned that when energy builds and the inner world calls out for attention, I need to take what I call "a healing vacation." Inwardly I feel drawn to retreat, and the message becomes very clear as to where I am supposed to go. Once I had left my daily life behind I had time to rest, fast, meditate, and experience solitude, so that I could focus my attention on my inner life. A few days later when I returned to my home and daily life, I was clear and ready to go on. This process worked well for me, but every woman's situation and process is different. Each woman must follow her own inner voice and guidance.

Once I could not leave Cambridge when I was processing something profoundly deep. As I did not want to be disturbed by my family responsibilities, I asked a woman friend if I could camp on her land over the weekend. Surrounded by the glory of her wild country garden, I fasted in solitude on lemon juice and water, meditated, slept and allowed my attention to sink deep inside. About noon on Sunday I became ill and began to vomit. My friend came running out and held me while my body convulsed, and then as I sobbed and cried. She laid me on a blanket and massaged me, comforting me and soothing me with songs and words and touch. When she had finished the massage, I asked her if I could put my head in her lap. She held me as if I were her child and I felt loved, understood and comforted. This friend was also menopausal. She had also left her husband and understood what I was going through. It was such a relief for me to allow someone to support me and mother me, I, who was support, practitioner and teacher to hundreds of students and patients. Tears of happiness flowed down my cheeks. We do not have to go far, or take trips of great expense, but we do need to get away, to retreat, to have the space to allow the energy and the emotional experience to surface and complete itself without distraction.

Creativity can open outrageous and wonderful solutions whenever there is a rise of energy, emotions like anger or fear, or even a physical symptom or illness. Once my communion with my inner ghostly lover (described in Jung's work as an imaginary divine figure that represents the masculine self which seeks integration and union with the feminine) became very powerful and demanded full attention. Because this experience was so intense, I arranged to take a week off, and got a last minute bargain flight to Morocco where I stayed in a seaside garden hotel in Agadir. Except for two walks along the ocean shore every day, I stayed in my room where I meditated and worked to clear this energy of illusion from my inner psyche. Another time when my fear was activated by severe slander, I went to a Buddhist monastery in the Lake District in the north of England, where I retreated into meditation and silence for five days, relieved only by long, solitary walks around the lake. By the end of this inspiring time I not only had received all the answers I needed, but I had achieved a state of compassionate detachment which completely changed my attitude to the slander. Once again, interior descent provided all that was required for me to deal with a challenge in my life.

When women consulted me with severe physical symptoms and emotional distress I would insist that they take a retreat for at least seven days. Once they did this, and returned and reported to me what had happened, I would agree to work with them. The retreat was an essential part of the healing process. That was the way they got in touch with their essential self again. Once they had done that, truth could begin to work again in their lives.

Aside from taking personal retreats to try to work with and clear the energy as it accumulated and rose to the surface, I also attempted to discuss what was happening to me with my husband, so that I could make him part of the process. However, not only was he completely oblivious that anything was happening to me, but he was impatient and distracted. He would not listen or give his attention, but would get up after a few minutes, saying that he was too busy to talk about such things. He had no interest in my inner reality or my thoughts and feelings. This behavior confirmed the truth about my decision to leave.

Consequently the depth of sadness and apathy increased. Nothing worked to bring me out of this state. Life seemed hopeless because I realized how imprisoned I was by the chains my previous martyr persona had created around me. I sought for a way to break this state and tried many things, but nothing worked. This depression went on for about six weeks, until one morning I woke up with one thought in my mind – to go to Delphi in Greece and visit the ancient sites of the priestesses who gave oracles to those who came seeking help, direction and understanding. I asked my secretary, Sue, if she would like to come with me, and of course her face lit up with a big yes. In less than a week we were in Athens. We rented a car and drove through the mountains which were fragrant with golden–yellow broom and spring wildflowers. That night on the eve of my forty–fourth birthday, after visiting the oracular pool and climbing the smooth worn steps into the ancient center of the world, I was given a visionary dream.

First I experienced myself standing with my hands above my head and behind my back. My hands were moving upward, very, very, very slowly, through infinite time and space towards something I could not see. As my arms finally reached the top of my head I saw a magnificent broadsword in my hands and felt tremendous weight as this sword slowly, ever so slowly, descended, the blade glittering and shining as it caught light in its jewels and carvings. Then, suddenly before me I saw a writhing ball of threads, a huge knot. Every string represented attachments, connections, karmas, all woven together as my English destiny – husband, children, home, neighbors, friends and hundreds of patients and students. Then the sword moved with a flash and descended cleanly and clearly to cut through the knot and the strings of light flew apart. The energy released created an explosion and I woke in the darkness shaking and excited by the beauty and truth of the dream. I came to Greece to visit the ancient oracular sites, seeking a solution, and one had been given to me, a true clearing within my own being.

The depression was gone. My Gordian knot had been cut. I was free to move on. Radiantly jubilant, I continued my pilgrimage to the ancient sites of Epidaurus and Eleusis. When I returned from Greece I told my husband I would be leaving him, and returning to America, and over the next few months this truth became reality. As karmas and destinies sorted themselves out, I moved my school and herb company from our large home outside Cambridge to a 16th century inn named Dolphin House, on Gold Street, in Saffron Walden, Essex, for the period of transition before I could wind up my affairs and leave England.

Although it was my deepest wish to separate peacefully and remain friends, this was not to be. As my husband experienced his own anger, attachment and grief he acted out his pain by hurting me, instead of taking responsibility for his own feelings. During this time my menstrual periods became more and more painful. As he became increasingly angry and violent on the outside, I tensed inside, harming my own body. The pains became worse and eventually I realized I was creating endometriosis.

Although my life situation was already difficult, more was yet to come. While I was on a short trip to India visiting my spiritual teacher, my husband contacted solicitors. When I returned home I discovered that he had moved my and my children's personal possessions out of our house and into the teaching room at the school. His legal counsel advised me that I could not go back into my home.

This betrayal was a deep shock and against everything we had mutually agreed upon. I plunged deeply into grief, waking up sobbing, bursting into tears several times a day and going to sleep sobbing. It was as though every wound and every sadness had collected in one place through this deep betrayal. When this excessive emotion dissolved at the end of three weeks I had developed acute pain in my knees. I couldn't walk properly and was no longer able to sit on my knees or cross–legged. I lived with the symptoms for a time, thinking they would go away. When they did not subside, I went to the Institute of Naturopathic and Yogic Sciences in Bangalore, India, for a three week purification and rejuvenation. During the consultation the doctor examined my knees, took X–rays and then advised me I had arthritis. I was shocked that an emotional upset could so quickly produce a severe illness. During my time there I underwent the deepest purification since I had healed breast cancer at twenty–five years of age.

At five o'clock on the eleventh day of a lemon water fast, which was supported by daily water therapies, herbal enemas, massage, steambaths, saunas, physiotherapy, mud treatments, yoga, pranayam, exercise and color therapy sunbaths, I experienced severe diarrhea, something very rare in my life, both in daily life or during purification. For five hours, until about ten o'clock, my bowels periodically cramped in spasms and released small black pellets of fecal matter. I was fine for the rest of the day, until about five o'clock the next morning, when the cycle repeated. I had thought my bowels were empty after so many days of fasting and enemas, but I was amazed at what came out of me. After three days of this healing crisis my legs were no longer swollen and painful, and the hard crystals in the tissues around my knees had disappeared. I could sit cross–legged again. The fasting and treatment were successful.

The healing process also included inner work on emotional, mental and spiritual levels to forgive my husband and to completely release the pain of my marriage, separation and divorce. If this too had not been accomplished, the condition would not have healed so completely, and it would have returned. Although I recovered from the arthritis, the endometriosis did not clear. I realized I needed a different approach to release the endometriosis and felt confident that I could heal the condition once the trauma of separation and divorce was over.

I do not like to think of what life would have been like if I had not been able to clear this out of my body, heart and mind and move on. Although my husband's behavior was a betrayal and a deep emotional wound, it showed me what I had always known instinctively, that he was not my friend. It also gave me the opportunity to detach completely and begin my own life. In the end I chose to let go of my home and the financial settlements that were due me. I refused to go to court and accepted the small amount he decided to give me because I knew entanglement with him over many months and perhaps years would not be good for me.

The process of menopause continued, and my entire life was changing all around me. The powerful energies of the change had wrought transformation. I was no longer the same person. Time passed, a difficult, painful time when every fiber of my being seemed stretched beyond capacity. Then the horizon opened. On a trip to a seminar in America I discovered and bought a beautiful dome on three acres in the Rocky Mountains. Difficult months of traveling back and forth, completing work with my English students and clients, selling leases and personal effects and packing, finally resulted in my move in February 1988 to Gold Hill, Boulder, Colorado.

I named my new home, *Wisdome*, because it was a bell shaped dome, a mountain temple, round with round windows, all curved inside. Living in it was like being on the inside of a lotus or a feminine spiritual womb that was symbolic of my menopausal transformation. I surrounded it with a mandalic deck that appeared in my inner eye as a vision, the design of which was formed from two vesica pisces (the feminine shape for receptivity to God), the squaring of the circle shape of the dome, and a medicine wheel aligned with the four directions, all contained within a flower petal design reminiscent of the muladhara earth root chakra. This sacred geometry deck symbolized my intent to ground my spiritual being in physical reality. My five years there were a most amazing and wonderful time. I treasured and made good use of the solitude, the peace and the creativity which flowed from my soul and my inner essence. I was amazed and grateful that the universe had provided me with a sanctuary which reflected my inner processes by its unique and beautiful architecture.

During that time menopause surfaced and faded away in cycles. Sometimes the change was physical, at other times, mental, emotional, sexual or spiritual. Always it was the same energy movement, a rise to the surface which demanded attention, release and completion which resulted in transformation. I had become at home with the process. If women would commune and work with these natural energies as they arise, and receive them as a creative priority, many problems would be avoided. Not only would they have amazing experiences, but they would open the energy flow, so that the work of healing and transformation could take place unhindered.

Women are essentially receptive in nature. For our first thirty–five to forty years we take the world into our being. Many women reach a saturation point around menopause where we cannot take in any more. We have to clear. We have to empty. We have to find our essence again. As we seek our truer deeper self we are forced to activate our animus, our internal masculine energy, which is necessary both to cut through the knot of our life and to help us achieve our goals. Usually we project this energy outside, infusing men with the power of our inner masculine, making them our gods, through romantic love and transference. Only our inner ghostly lover can be our ideal perfect mate, but this state of perfection exists only in our imagination. We have to cut through this illusion, reach a union of masculine and feminine within, and come to a ground of balanced reality where we are complete within ourselves and do not demand that our partners reflect our ideals of perfection. Once we have achieved this, sexuality and relationships change, encompassing an equality and freedom we were never able to achieve before. We can truly enjoy being ourselves, and we can allow and support men to be themselves. We are finally ripe for a relationship of true compassionate, unconditional love balanced within by the divine inner marriage.

Although it may not always seem so when we are caught in the threads of pain and despair, there is always a creative approach to work with these energetic transformations. Yet, so many women repress, deny, ignore, or refuse to make changes. They won't let go, and choose to suffer instead. I discovered that whenever I took the time away from my daily life to focus on what was happening within me, the energy released and I attained a new level of self–realization. Once this had been experienced a few times, confidence developed. The journey became exciting instead of scary. I began to enjoy the process, looking forward to the next surge and enjoying the opportunity to cooperate with this raw elemental energy seeking release and transformation. This energy is intense, beyond form, potent and pure. It is released from the essence and roots of our being to help us achieve transformation.

After the move from England to Colorado, there was a great shift in my menopausal experience. I had burst free and now I wanted to celebrate. I began to dance. There high in the mountains, inside and outside my mountain home, *Wisdome*, I danced like a goddess, alone and with sisters, students and friends, in the spring and summer in my exquisite flowering meadow, in the winter snow in blizzards, in the light of the full moon as it created a circle through the large round window of my dome, under the stars and before God. I danced and danced and could not get enough of this dancing. It was as though I were creating my own form. I searched for and bought music, and explored movement, vibration, and making shapes and rhythms with my body. The dancing was my greatest healing during menopause. I danced out my emotional wounds, my pelvic tension and the endometriosis. It was how my being chose to integrate all the different aspects of my life, reconnect with nature and harmonize the elements of life. My dances eventually developed into the Elemental Energetics workshops that I share in seminars in England, America, South Africa, Australia, Malaysia and India.

I made several more trips to India to the feet of my spiritual teacher where I danced in my room between the satsangs, expressing my happiness and my gratitude for the gift of His love. When He passed from this world my grief was boundless and after two months of intense longing, I took a trip to Kauai in the Hawaiian islands where I swam in the tropical waters. My play in the ocean released me from the chains of grief and life went on once again.

Period irregularities came and went. My hair began to turn silver. I went through a few bouts of exhaustion after returning from international teaching trips. After one six–week episode of fatigue after an English summer school, I realized it was time to take a break. I rented out my dome, turned the school over to my daughter, Casel, and traveled through Hawaii to Malaysia. I then spent four months in India where I took a four–week purification at the Institute of Naturopathic and Yogic Sciences, stayed a month at my ashram near Beas in the Punjab, and visited friends in Jaipur and in the Himalayas. I returned home via Hawaii, enjoying another two week tropical holiday. This trip was one of the most wonderful things I ever did for myself. I came home completely well, rested and rejuvenated. There was no point trying to fit myself back into an old shell, so I got to work. Changes needed to be made once again.

I now felt a call to live more simply. I gave away and sold many possessions. As much as I loved the splendid isolation of my mountain home, I knew I needed to move down into the Boulder community. My cycle of reclusiveness was over, and it was time to find an apartment in town, walk everywhere, have a low overhead and write my books. I followed my instincts, let go and moved on to the next phase.

I enjoy the freedom of being single and have always appreciated the resources that are available to me, so that I can travel, take retreats and leave my daily life from time to time to process my inner life. Any woman can do this within her own circumstances. There is always a way. North American Indian women used to pack up their bedrolls and camp out, go on vision quests, and retreat into moon lodges. Healing centers and women's groups are now providing sanctuaries for the feminine experience. Women have to find the courage to take themselves away. What they bring back to their lives will benefit everyone and everything. We are not being selfish. We are following the ancient sacred golden path of the feminine. The temple of the spirit within must be nourished.

When health problems occur, I apply my creative medicine woman energy to the challenge; I have worked through and freed myself from spinal problems, gum disease, irregular periods, fatigue, falling hair, digestive upsets and stress. I always ask myself questions. How have I created this? Why has my body chosen to react in this way? What is my body trying to tell me? I track down the cause, treat it, change my living habits, and clear spiritual, mental, or emotional resistances. In every case I do not let the problem continue once I am aware of it. I make it a priority so that it will not take over my life or give me a bigger problem later. Sometimes I seek the help of other natural practitioners, massage therapists, acupuncturists, polarity therapists, chiropractors or osteopaths. I never consult a medical practitioner, other than to have a routine pap smear, which is always clear. I take herbs regularly, fast once or twice a year, exercise as much as possible and live a moderate and simple lifestyle. Although emotional or mental reactions to people and events in my destiny result in health crises from time to time, my daily life habits are preventive, so symptoms heal quickly. As time passes my reactions become less and less and my experience of life is happier and easier.

During the spring of 1993 I planted an herb garden outside my front door and used my monthly blood to water the plants. I let out the blood into a container, mixed it with water and laughed as I poured this magic pink fluid into the earth surrounding my plants. What a wonderful garden! The fragrance of the plants made me happy every day. I placed my garden chair near them, so I could enjoy eating or having cups of herbal tea while I sat with my plants. Every time I had a period I was sure it would be my last one. Then another would appear, and I would rejoice and celebrate as if this one would be my last. With pauses, they still come. I am looking forward to planting a new garden, this spring of 1994, with the blood from my womb.

The more I clear the thorns and weeds from my life, the more space there is for the roses, lilies and lotuses of my heart's dreams to bloom. I experience love and happiness in daily life in a way I never dreamed possible. I live in the present, in a place of abundant giving and receiving. I speak and live the truth. Waves of karmas come and I work them through and go on; always constant is my devotion to my meditation and my spiritual path.

Now I am enjoying the realization of a life–long dream, the creation of a book on women's, medicine, *Creative Menopause – Illuminating Women's Health and Spirituality*. Through the years I have also kept a *Diary of Blood*, a record of my moon cycle memories during menopause, which I hope to share in the future. Now at the completion of my menopausal cycle, nearly ten years since the first hot flashes, it is a great honor to write this book. It is my wish that this book be given life in this world to serve and inspire all women who share this amazing journey.

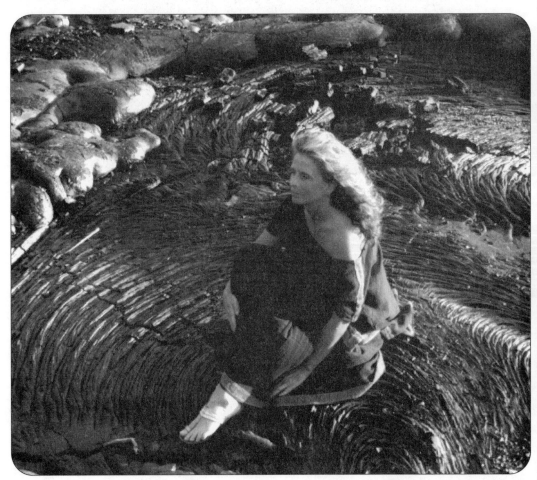

*Farida on lava flows, Hawaii, 1993*

# Life Cycles of the Feminine

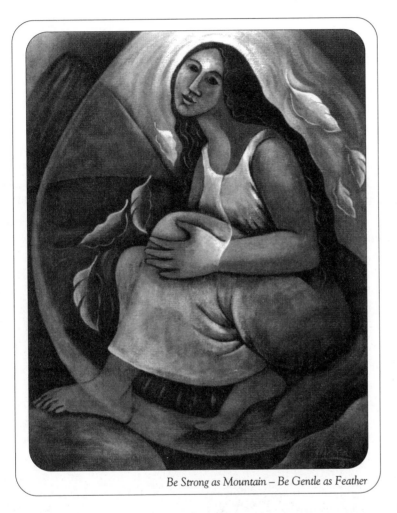

*Be Strong as Mountain – Be Gentle as Feather*

By the time we reach mid-life women have passed through many transitions. We have grown from a female infant into a young girl, and flowered into a maiden, wife, lover or mother. Not everyone will experience each role. Some will experience other transitions into students, academics, workers, professionals, artists, business owners and other possibilities, both negative and positive. We also experience wounds that deepen our lives as well as challenge us. Women celebrate their departures from old roles and their entrances into new roles, but rarely do we celebrate mid-life or menopause. Aging is regarded fearfully. Energy is directed towards preserving youth, rather than developing the beauty, wisdom and spirituality of our elder years. Very little is done to prepare for this major change, and many women come to this time depleted, disenchanted and without any realistic information or guidance.

Menopause is not something we should shrink from. We should look forward to it, prepare for it and rejoice when it arrives. We should share it with our family, our friends and our world. Women have kept silent for too long. We must bring our inner feeling level to the surface where it can be healed, transformed and given strength and purpose. We are the raw ore and we are the gold. The creativity is with our own life energy, within our own body. There is a great opportunity for us to birth ourself into the next cycle of our life. How we have lived our life up to the time that we enter menopause creates the ground for the experience that we will have, and the depth and breadth of the opportunity for completion, integration and transformation. Let us look at what we can do at the different stages of our life, so that we are fully prepared for our mid-life opportunity.

Once we begin our menstrual cycle at menarche during puberty and begin to move through our reproductive years towards menopause, our hormones regulate different aspects of our monthly cycle, but are we really aware of what is taking place in our body? Personally, I was not aware of changes during my cycle for many years, and I never felt ovulation taking place until I was in my early thirties. All the eggs are present in the foetus at the end of the second trimester, and we carry them within us, releasing them monthly, until they are gone. The mystery of our reproductive systems seems beyond understanding. We can try to explain it with science or we can dissect women's bodies. Only women know what these processes feel like in their bodies.

For years I could not understand what a hormone was. The words and concepts had no meaning or reality for me. I never saw a picture of estrogen, and when I asked a medical doctor exactly what estrogen was, I was told that what is commonly named estrogen was made up of over two dozen steroidal hormones. For me, interior visualization and my life experience was more real than a medical name of a hormone which didn't really exist except as a concept. I finally established a relationship with my hormones when I experienced an inner vision of my endocrine organs. I realized they were connected with both cosmic planetary forces in the outer world and subtle chakra and elemental energies within my own being. Once I had visualized their connectedness with the inner and outer universes, I was able to experience hormones as exquisite crystals that reflected their unique vibratory resonance. These shapes were stimulated by other crystals within the body and influenced by crystalline forces in the universe. Within whatever individual process is personally valuable and truthful, women need to tune in to their own bodies and take the time to understand and experience for themselves what hormones are, what they do and how they influence our body, mind and emotions. We need to take the information out of our head and into our experience.

There are different types of hormones which trigger different parts of our cycle, different crystalline messengers which stimulate the cycles of birthing the egg, preparing the womb and releasing the blood. From the first day of our cycle to ovulation we birth an egg in our ovary during the follicular phase. Once we ovulate and the egg comes down the fallopian tube into the uterus, we are in the luteal progesterone phase of fertility that increases the lining of the uterus in anticipation of fertilization, until the monthly flow releases the lining, or we become pregnant. These rising and falling tides within our womb reflect the ebb and flow of the oceanic tides in response to the waxing and waning of the moon.

If we are fully aware of our body, we feel different during each part of our cycle, unless we take the pill which neutralizes this process. Instead of alternating between estrogen and progesterone cycles synthetic hormones flatten and control our monthly cycles. When we experience pre–menstrual symptoms, truth is being revealed about the condition of our lives. Whatever we have not taken care of physically, emotionally or mentally manifests before and during our monthly flow, when the veil between the seen and the unseen, and the outer and inner world thins. If we do not take this monthly opportunity to experience truth, develop our wisdom and make positive changes in our life, these repressed truths submerge, collect and stagnate in our unconscious. Eventually this negativity manifests in the physical body with strong messages of symptoms, distress and disease that cannot be denied. We may be able to put truth off for a while, but we pay the price by having a greater problem to deal with later on.

Everything we do in this world has a price. Whatever choice we make determines our future. If we use the pill it will affect our body and our hormones. Women in their forties and fifties are now experiencing the results of the pill's effect on their menopause. I could never take the pill. It made me vomit. I could only tolerate an IUD for twelve hours before I had to have it taken out. My body has never been controlled by synthetic hormones or implants and I believe this has helped me to experience my authentic being during a positive, healthy and creative mid–life transition.

Women's cycles are meant to be more than a physical experience. Along with the oceanic tides and the ebb and flow of blood, our emotions rise and fall. Rather than neutralize this aspect of our femininity with the pill in order to please men, or avoid pregnancy, we must find the strength to seek and find male companions, lovers and husbands who will honor the feminine instead of using and abusing it. We must also elevate sexuality, and experience the more subtle, cosmic and tantric aspects of union that do not put us at risk from pregnancy. From menarche, when we begin our monthly flow, through all our experiences of female sexuality, we need to preserve and protect our wombs and respect our moon cycles.

When we have our monthly flows it is fruitful and nourishing to cocoon, rest, be alone, think, dream, go inside, and restore and refresh ourselves. Primitive women secluded themselves in their moon lodges to create the opportunity to communicate with their inner lives and receive guidance, visions and clarity. Modern women need to slow down, appreciate and honor our cyclic nature that serves the purpose of nourishing the feminine. In goal–oriented modern life human beings tend to override this cyclic aspect of their lives and they and the world suffer as a result. Each woman's contribution to this planetary dilemma is significant. As each woman changes, the world changes.

Women often ovulate or have their periods on the full moon or the new moon. When women live together their cycles synchronize naturally. The new moon period is yin, or receptive, and the full moon period is yang and creative – yet in the fullness of one is the seed of the other. A new moon ovulation is inward and feminine, and a full moon ovulation is more receptive to sexuality and fertilization by the male. These alternating cycles are in rhythm with the universe. Within this rising and falling, conception, the ultimate creative event, celebrates the boundless fertility of this cosmos.

We need to awaken our sensitivity to the moon cycles. We can purchase calendars which display the moon cycles and record our ovulation and monthly flow on them. We can also draw the moon cycles onto our calendars and in our diaries. Consider the time of the monthly flow when making appointments. Look at the moon in the sky and watch its changes. Become aware of ovulation and the womb filling with blood. Feel the moon, the cycles and the tides within the body. Prepare for each monthly flow and allow time and space to experience their depth and potential vision of truth.

If we become deeply involved in our preparation for menopause it is important that we safeguard and preserve the continued healthy function of the liver, the bowels, the adrenals and the lymphatic system. These organs and glands are directly concerned with the menopause experience. We need to develop an understanding of natural health and our own unique strengths and weaknesses. We also want to know how to utilize simple remedies, dietary support and home therapeutics to help us through any minor illnesses instead of suppressing conditions and using over–the–counter or prescription drugs. If we don't take time to support and nourish our boies, they will make us take the time by presenting us eventually with a major illness crisis. If we don't learn to stop, the universe will stop us.

Women often deplete themselves in their twenties and thirties as they expend their energies in relationships, marriages, homemaking, careers and childrearing. Modern 'life–on–the–run' can be a recipe for disaster. Stressful lifestyles deplete calcium which is so essential for menopause. We must take care to take enough organic calcium during our twenties and thirties, especially during pregnancy and nursing, so that we are not calcium deficient as we enter mid–life. We also need to take natural calcium before and during our menopause transition to prepare for the five–year bone growth pause which follows the cessation of the monthly flows. If we prepare well, we can avoid osteoporosis, or bone loss.

Today many women realize that they need a support system. Instead of being separated from other women because of sexual and professional competition and cultural isolation in communities, homes and apartments, more and more women take the time today to join together in groups, sweat lodges, workshops and retreats. Women now work in professions which were once male dominated, giving other women the choice to seek and find a woman doctor, lawyer, engineer, banker or accountant. Women's magazines, and newspapers continue to multiply. Women's health and spirituality are the subjects of rapidly growing markets in literature, media, music, videos and art. We are reaching out to each other in every way and building both a practical and a visionary net of communication and support. The earlier we build our personal network, the more support we will have during our menopause, and the easier it will be to share our experience, to learn from other women who have passed through their transition, and to make the most of the challenge of our creative menopausal passage.

As women begin to explore and define their inner worlds it is only natural that our spirituality will unfold. Today there are many ways that women can access their inner worlds and develop a relationship with their higher Self and the divine. There are strong movements of growth in the New Age areas of healing, channeling, ancient mysteries, oracles, storytelling, sacred psychology, and in the more traditional disciplines of yoga, tai chi and meditation. In the past few years there has been a marked increase in women gurus and spiritual teachers, some of them manifesting as incarnations of the Divine Mother. Our hearts and minds may lead us to explore and experience different teachers and different paths, and when it is appropriate to move on, it is important we let go and return to the search. Because spirituality is a natural aspect of menopause, women are drawn to face this deeper level of their being. We need to follow wherever that stream of attraction may lead and let the vibration of our longing meet and resonate with our spiritual destiny.

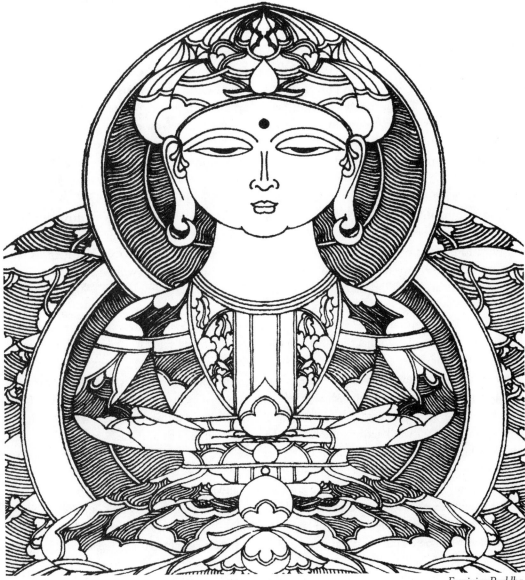

*Feminine Buddha*

Because today's world–mind creates a very powerful media reality, glamorizing beauty products, fashion, homes, computers, automobiles, travel, and household gadgetry, many women end up buying things instead of creating them, and working at jobs they may not like just to fulfill their expected role as a consumer. While the rest of the world may envy our material success and abundant lifestyles, we need to realize how shallow and unsatisfactory this double–bind can be. Women must pull back into their inner beings and find out who they are, separate from the choices they make as workers or consumers.

It is very difficult to become free of our present–day culture. We may have to live in this culture, but we do not need to be driven by it. There is enough space and freedom in this world to create an authentic lifestyle that will support our highest purpose, so that we can live from our fountain of inner truth and creativity. Our lives become our greatest creation. We must take the time to find out who we are and then bring that truth into our lives and all that we do. When we become authentic we will find reflections everywhere that will support and nourish the truth of our lives. This creative, mystical process is at its height during menopause. It is as though the universe is saying, "This is the time to truly become yourself. You can't put it off any longer."

We must take time for our inner lives, get to know ourselves, experience deep rest and rejuvenation, and spend time doing what nourishes us. Retreats support our mid–life transformation by providing opportunities for solitude and inner attention. If we take an interest in our health during our youth we will have fewer nettles, thorns and thistles to cause us pain, illness and suffering in our menopausal harvest. We should live with respect for our bodies instead of using them up as we live the fast life, burn the candle at both ends, or drive ourselves in pursuit of success, status and material goals. If we are interested in building a healthy lifestyle we need to prevent problems by establishing a dialogue with our bodies that will help us take care of ourselves. If we have ignored health realities for forty years it will be more difficult to achieve physical and emotional health when we are in the vulnerable and sensitive time of menopause.

Solitude is essential to our menopause years. We find peace by giving ourselves the space to be still, so that we can connect with our spirituality. For many years we have lived within the whirlwind of our desires, duties and responsibilities, and now we must go deeper to the core of our being that is beyond activity and beyond desire. The modern world is increasingly involutionary, or outward. Women are seduced by the media into becoming more outward and active. Because this is in contradiction to their esential nature, this leads to disease. Cycles of both inward and outward activity are essential for personal growth and the balance of the male and female energies. Yet many women no longer take the time to let go of worldly activities and connect with their inner selves. This is the challenge. This is what is needed for balance. We have become conditioned to believe the answers are outward. Now is the time to change.

Menopause is our time to connect with and establish a relationship with our deeper selves. It is a time to gather strength for our elder years and our transition out of our bodies, our lives and this world. The earlier we begin to take personal retreats the more prepared we will be when our change of life begins. If we are already comfortable with our inner lives, we will be able to take up the challenge, enjoy the transition and experience our own creative mid–life transition.

# Diamond Menopause

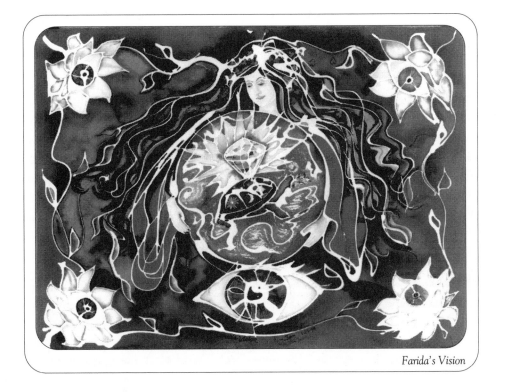

*Farida's Vision*

The different facets of menopause may seem unrelated when we separate them for the purpose of exploration, definition and reference. The opportunity of the Diamond Menopause is clearly the integration of physical, emotional, mental and spiritual aspects of our being. Each facet affects every other facet, and is affected by every other facet. Together they form a personal holistic life ecology. No facet must be left neglected, unconscious or unborn. We must strive with our entire being to become our fullest possible greatest self, a fully awakened true human being. We must believe that we can attain self realization and God realization as this is the highest purpose of our life.

We have a choice whether to focus on what is aging and fading, or on what is growing and evolving. This choice creates our experience of the mid–life transition and our departure from our body, our life and this world. The outward physical flowering of our womanhood, our youth and our feminine beauty will fade, but we can become illuminated by a greater beauty, the radiance of our spiritual diamond beauty of integration that shines from within. If we lose ourselves in physical, emotional and mental menopause, without receiving nourishment and inspiration from our spirituality, then it will be harder to let go of our identification with youth and beauty. Our experience will be one of uncomfortable resistance. If we focus on the spiritual and awaken to the divine bliss and love within, this will enable us to effortlessly release what is passing away. Just like the petals that unfurl from the center of a flower, we need to allow what is fading to fertilize the phoenix flower of our transformation and move more deeply into the potency and power of the seed force that contains both our essence and our future.

Physical menopause is often the most obvious because it is something that we can see, feel, taste, touch, hear and sense. We have a pain. We have a symptom. Our body functions change. We don't feel right. We ask for help. When we are suffering, we are vulnerable. We are full of fear. We most often don't know what to do, or where to turn for help. Suddenly the life that we have been living comes to a halt, or has to be adjusted. We need to take time to seek professional advice. We have to use money to pay for consultations, treatments, surgery and drugs, or alternative, preventive, and therapeutic education and care.

The purpose of these pains and symptoms is to awaken us. Our bodies are calling out for help. They have been ignored too long. We begin our healing journey when we try to find a way out of the situation we have created. What price will we pay? What choices will we make? How will our life stories turn out? It is up to us.

We learn that our physical problems are related to our emotions, our mind, our spirit and the way that we have lived our lives. There are books, cassettes, videos, workshops and television programs that teach this holistic approach, but how do we put this information into practical use in our own lives? When we have life–threatening conditions, our dear ones fear that they will lose us, so they urge us toward drastic medical approaches. Doctors try to rush us into decisions before we can think about what we are agreeing to and before we can try other methods.

It is a big commitment to take all this on at once, this self–healing, this descent into one's depths and this potential for transformation. The physical often leads us into all the other realms, and as we give energy to the process, our lives unfold toward integration. There is tremendous energy within us that wishes to support this process. If we tune in and flow with this energy instead of responding with fear and resistance, it will take us where we need to go.

Emotional menopause can be dramatic. Emotional excesses and passions may frighten the men in our lives, embarrass our friends and families, endanger our work and social status, and cause inner turmoil, yet medical doctors tell women that this experience is all 'in their mind' and prescribe tranquilizers and sedatives. Hysterectomies were invented by male doctors who believed that the emotional excesses of women would be relieved by removal of the uterus. This is simply not true. Women contain and repress the secrets of what they endure within themselves and injure their reproductive organs in the process. The physical damage may be removed surgically, but the emotions themselves do not arise from the uterus, but from an inability to integrate our life experience. That is the true work that needs to be accomplished.

During mid–life our emotions seek truthful release and expression because we can no longer contain ourselves or be contained. Energy is disruptive by nature because it must move, change and transform everything it is a part of and everything around it. This is the process of a conscious mid–life passage. Truth cannot be held back any longer. However, there are positive means of working with and supporting the emotional releases without being violent or destructive, and these methods are discussed in the Emotional Clearing section.

Sexuality is totally intertwined with the mid–life experience because it is an expression of our entire being – physical, emotional, mental and spiritual. In many ways menopause is a sexual experience, one that moves us out of personal sexuality into cosmic sexuality. Energies that were directed toward attracting a mate and bringing children into the world are now expanding towards self exploration, service, release from this physical world, spirituality and divine union.

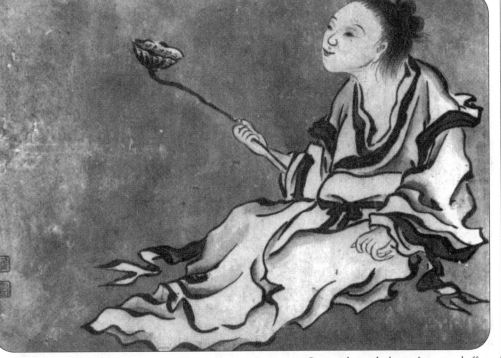

*Contemplating the lotus of cause and effect*

One of my patients who went through several months of purification, regeneration and transformation to successfully clear cervical dysplasia, experienced a powerful vision during a bodywork session toward the completion of her healing process. During the session she became aware of how she was limiting her sexuality, even though she had a happy and loving relationship with her husband and family. When she opened her internal vision she experienced a spiritual awakening of cosmic sexuality, expressing itself with exquisite flowerings of lotuses in the subtle bodies surrounding her sexual organs together with visions of goddesses and iridescent colors. She emerged from this session with an expanded vision that allowed her access to the creative healing movement of universal life energy. If we do not allow this expansion, our energy is spent in contraction and inhibition that contributes to physical difficulties and diminishes our ability to receive and allow healing. Her medical doctor told her that healing such an advanced cancerous condition in the cervix with natural medicine was impossible. However, when the medical tests came back the tissues were normal.

Mental winnowing requires pulling out the roots of our negativity, pruning wild growth that we have left unchecked, and nourishing the positive aspects of our being, so that our life may blossom like a garden warmed by the sun of our spirituality. Because we can no longer ignore the fruits of our thoughts and actions, we must be willing to look at the truth, clear the weeds from the garden of our lives, and sow new seeds for the future. During mid–life we are forced to experience the fruits of previous thoughts and actions, so it is essential that we clear the past as well as sow new seeds. Purification and regeneration must proceed together, so that transformation can unfold naturally.

Spirituality opens when we long for the higher life and when our heart and soul are attracted only to love. Just as we look for a teacher when we wish to learn, we need to seek for a spiritual adept who is both a living example and a guide. If we call out from the depths of our being, spirituality will open for us, but soul life is not to be achieved by manipulation or goal–oriented activities. It requires surrender of what we are to something greater. We need to leave our personal selves behind in order to gain the greater Self. It is not the letting go that we should focus on, but what we are receiving. The more we practice letting go of our personal selves, the easier it is to receive the divine impulse, enabling us to prepare for the highest role of our elder years, that of spiritual preparation for our passage from this world to higher levels of God consciousness.

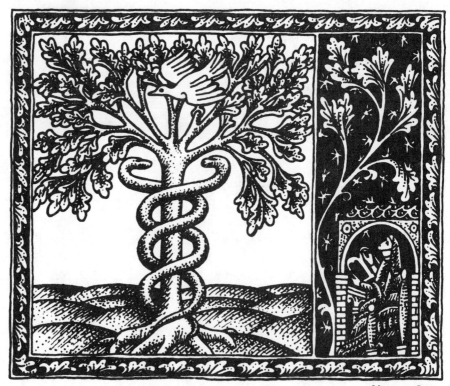

*Visionary Scene*

# *Physical Healing*

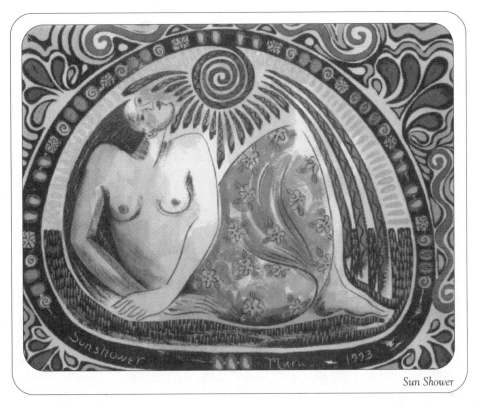

*Sun Shower*

Spinning straw into gold is the work of mid–life and menopause. We must transform negativity into positivity. Excellent health can be won by correct living and natural healing, even during mid–life. If the physical cannot be totally rejuvenated, pain can be lessened and our passing eased. The gold can also be realized in emotional, mental and spiritual realms. We must have the courage and the vision to realize that just as we created weakness and disease through our life experience and our habits, we can also create strength and health.

It can be hard to find our way as women in these modern times. There are so many influences and pressures. We are not a culture that shows us a positive way with myth, metaphor, tradition and ritual. We do not have rites of initiation which pass on the wisdom of our mothers and our mother's mothers. We are also expected to remain women while we perform like men in the work world. The stresses are enormous.

Each woman must find her unique path. We can either live as a reflection of the expectations of others or develop our interior, intuitive wisdom and instincts which will guide us to know what is right. While this may seem difficult, especially when we are so out of touch with ourselves, it is the claiming of that instinctive feminine nature that will prove a center of strength in a changing, confusing, and constantly overstimulating world.

We learn we cannot rely on external sources of information, no matter how authoritative they seem, to guide us in our health choices. We pay the price in our own bodies for whatever choices we make. We must learn how to tune in to our inner knowing. The path to a healthy female body lies in understanding individual strengths and weaknesses, having a stable emotional life, living a moderate natural lifestlye and keeping the eliminative systems active. While it is true that life creates stress and unexpected events, and our archetypal patterns and karmic patterns lead us into destinies and reactions that create health problems, it is the work of maturity to learn to ride the waves of life so that we do not harm ourselves.

The signs of illness are there far in advance for us to recognize if we pay attention. However, many women shrug these advance warnings aside due to the pressures of family and work responsibilities, and from ignorance or fear. These warnings, if ignored, develop eventually into chronic disease patterns. The healing process requires that the knot of mind/emotion/body causes be released.

Much of what threatens women is centered around the reproductive system. Methods of contraception, birth practices and radical surgery are great stress areas for women. We have become dependent on a technology that we fear, resist and do not understand. How can we find the way out, and the way back to wisdom and understanding? How can we make our bodies our own again? The first steps are to feel, to listen and to pay attention. When there are changes or symptoms we must do something about them right away. Observe. Look for changes in bowels and urine, new facial lines, pains or undue fatigue. Instead of dulling the pain, accepting the pain and denying what is happening, we must center on our life and seek understanding. Read books. Find a natural physician. Become a part of support groups. Attend lectures and seminars. Establish a network of support and communication. Be willing to look at mental and emotional distress as the cause of physical ailments. Know that life is a progression. Even if there have not been women of wisdom to guide us, we can learn by experience and from each other, and eventually become a guide for younger women. Our mature years will have a purpose and a vision to which we can look forward.

The healing of menopausal attitudes and emotions is meant to be integrated with physical treatment. I also recommend that those who are interested in self–health–fulfillment receive an iridology analysis from a skilled practitioner to help them understand their unique constitutional type. Once they understand their strengths and weaknesses, they can consciously work toward achieving healing and balanced bodily function. The remedies and suggestions given for menopausal conditions will only be partially effective if the individual is not prepared to make positive changes with diet, lifestyle and eliminative activation. Refer to *Herbs of Grace – Becoming Independently Healthy* for information on herbal formulae, nutrition, home treatments, and detailed instructions on how to approach purification, regeneration and transformation.

It is important to understand that each person's body is completely unique. Individual strengths and weaknesses are affected by mind, emotions, stress, diet, lifestyle, constitution and destiny. Because symptoms, illnesses and problems emerge out of different combinations of weaknesses in the body systems, glands and organs, we will review the importance and function of each of the body systems and relate them to the change of life experience.

# BODY SYSTEMS, ORGANS & GLANDS

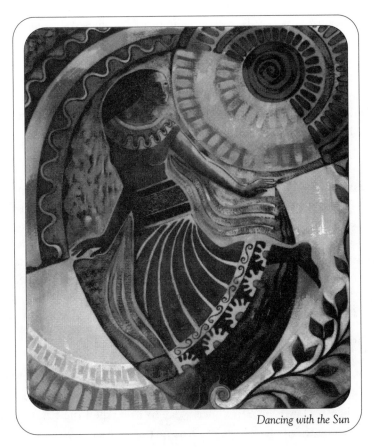

*Dancing with the Sun*

## CIRCULATORY SYSTEM

As we age our circulatory system slows down, unless we exercise regularly and keep the river of life flowing to all areas of our bodies. We need to make sure that the bowels, liver and lymphatic systems do their part to keep our blood clean. Menopause will be easier when the heart is receiving clear, clean blood to circulate throughout the body and the extremities. Memory, dizziness, inability to concentrate and circulatory problems can be avoided.

### Arteries

Hardening of the arteries is a common aging ailment caused by constitutional weakness, poor diet, thyroid imbalances, calcium imbalances and liver dysfunction. Arterial problems are reflections of excess activity and stressful outward moving energy. This condition requires full systemic treatment. Refer to the Circulatory Hardening constitutional type in *Herbs of Grace*.

### Heart

Heart disease is the number one cause of death in women. Diet plays a large part in creating this disease as does negativity and depression. The heart becomes stressed by ever–thickening blood that is struggling to move through narrowing, hardening arteries. Blood pressure changes and imbalances can also affect and stress the heart. Because the liver and the lymphatic system play an important role in cleaning the blood, it is essential to support their continued healthy function. Emotional wounding also influences the heart, creating depression and hopelessness. Instead of giving love we wait for someone to love us. If there is a lack of love it is because we will not love. We have chosen to focus on what we do not have, instead of what we have.

### Veins

Varicose veins cause great suffering to women during pregnancy and aging. While some constitutional types are prone to this condition, others create it though poor diet, stress and lack of self care. It is essential to treat this condition naturally at the earliest stages. Vein problems reflect a 'return to the source' stress. Full systemic treatment is required to increase the strength of the circulation, purify the blood and adjust spinal and postural problems. Massage, reflexology, baths, and fomentations soaked in Witch Hazel and Periwinkle infusions are effective aids.

## NATURAL TREATMENTS FOR THE CIRCULATORY SYSTEM

*Diet*: Avoid fats, fried foods, eggs, cholesterol and alcohol.

*Herbs*: Use the Blood Purifying, Circulation Systemic, Circulation Cerebral and Heart formulae; use liver and lymphatic herbs and formulae to support the circulatory system and to improve the quality of blood; chew a Hawthorn berry once a day to strengthen the heart; drink Buckwheat herbal infusion; take one teaspoon or more of Cayenne pepper each day.

*Therapies*: Exercise, walk and swim regularly; have a weekly massage and reflexology treatment; practice gentle, low impact aerobics; if you wish to avoid senility, poor memory and lack of ability to focus and concentrate, it is essential to keep the blood moving to the brain; avoid smoking and living in polluted areas; open your heart to give and receive love; enjoy service; take the time to enjoy being in the present moment.

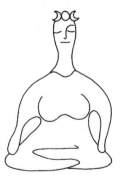

# DIGESTIVE SYSTEM

A disordered digestion lays the ground for many potential illnesses. All our body systems, organs and glands are dependent on the digestive system for nutrients and energy. We have to consider each part of the digestive tract, its contribution to body function and how any malfunction affects menopause. Whenever you feel congestion, pain or symptoms, your body is telling you it is time to pay attention, make changes and seek healing.

The digestive system is the home of the fire element presented in the Emotional Clearing section. The correlation of physical symptoms with emotional and mental influences is important because it helps us clear and integrate the causes of physical problems.

## Mouth, Teeth, Tongue, Tonsils, Lower Jaw

The journey of nourishment begins with what we put in our mouth, how it affects our taste buds, which cause reflex actions in our stomach, and how we chew and swallow. The condition of our gums and teeth as we age is determined to a large extent by the bacterial climate we have created in our gastrointestinal tract, our dental care habits and the nutrients we are able to absorb and utilize. Gums and teeth suffer when calcium is depleted by stress, and poor eating and living habits. Once problems develop it is difficult and expensive to overcome them.

## Esophagus and Trachea

Our throat swallows the food and drink we choose to nourish our body. If the food has been well chosen and chewed thoroughly in a relaxed and pleasant way, swallowing begins our process of digestive chemistry. As mid–life is a time to evaluate and upgrade our relationship with nourishment, we need to give time and attention to developing good eating habits.

## Stomach, Pylorus

How the food is digested in the stomach depends on how well it has been chewed. It is important not to dilute digestive juices with fluids, or to slow down digestion with iced drinks. Lower estrogen levels together with liver overloading due to increased levels of hormones being processed through the liver, also inhibit digestive processes. We have to learn to eat less, more slowly and with more care during the change of life. The world is yang, acid and active. We have to create a yin, alkaline and quiet inner world to balance the effects of the outer world.

## Duodenum

In the mixing chamber of the duodenum, the food from the stomach receives alkaline juices from the liver and the gall bladder, and acid juices from the pancreas. A balanced blending of acid and alkaline determines how well the food will be utilized in the small and large intestines. When there is stress, ulcers may occur in this area. Nourishment is an important aspect of mid–life because it is in our later years that poor dietary habits reap their effect. We have to implement new dietary habits that will sustain us during the change of life as well as help us to prevent further problems.

## Liver

This organ is very important during mid–life. The liver breaks down hormones so that the products of this process are made available for the production of new hormones. During menopause the liver struggles to deal with increasing quantities of luteinizing and follicle stimulating hormones. Therefore the liver is not so available for digestive processes. Constant eating congests the liver and diminishes its ability to function well. The liver is also affected by firey emotions such as anger, jealousy and frustration, which may be released during the mid–life change. A healthy liver brings joy, laughter and happiness to life, and provides clarity for long–range planning. An efficiently functioning liver also helps to preserve good eyesight.

## Gall Bladder

The assistant to the liver, the gall bladder, is also affected by anger. Gall stones can develop when strong fears crystallize on the physical level. Adequate levels of bile are necessary for healthy digestive functions, so it is important to keep this organ active and healthy.

## Small Intestines

These digestive organs are where, the Chinese say, "the pure is separated from the impure." Ideally, the small intestines are where nutrients are absorbed and processed, and the residue moved on into the large intestines for elimination. This function represents a very important aspect of menopause because this is our time to look at every aspect of our lives and make choices about what we will keep in our life and what we will release. Because mid–life is a time for letting go of what is self destructive or what no longer serves us, the energy of the small intestines resonates with this nourishment selection process. We need to know what is good for us and make sure that we give it to ourselves, and we need to release the rest.

## Ileocecal Valve

This valve connects the small and large intestines. It also determines when it is appropriate to release the food matter being processed from the small intestines into the colon. Strongly affected by emotions and stress, this valve is affected by tension in the psoas muscle in the abdomen. If food matter is let into the colon too soon, it will have too much fluid in it and will cause loose bowels. If it is held in the small intestines too long it becomes too dry, producing constipation. If there is congestion and constriction at the bottom of the ascending colon, and the appendix is not secreting sufficient antiseptic fluids, efforts need to be made to clear this area through Castor oil packs, massage and stress management. It is wise to seek help from body workers, kineseologists and chiropractors to help release this area and to understand the importance of the mind–emotion–body dynamic.

## Cecum, Appendix

This container area at the bottom of the ascending colon receives the food matter which has passed through the ileocecal valve. If it collects, the appendix stimulates lubricants to help its movement up the ascending colon and also secretes antiseptics which help prevent infection. When the appendix, a valuable part of our immune system, is removed this function is impaired.

It is important for menopausal women to have regular bowel movements and to avoid infection, inflammation, or the increase of toxins in the pelvis. It is essential that all parts of the immune system be kept at optimum function to help prevent reproductive disease. I advise all women to read and study *Herbs of Grace* and put the herbal and naturopathic procedures into practice, improve their dietary habits and prevent bowel problems.

## Large Intestines

The colon absorbs nutrients to be released into the blood and lymph for absorption and utilization. Avoid constipation. Keep your colon clean and regular. Bowels should move a minimum of two times a day. Active peristalsis is essential to avoid toxins being spread from the colon into the blood and lymph, causing further overload to the liver and the immune system. Bowel pockets in the transverse colon affect mental abilities, influence negative states of mind, cause fatigue, headaches, insomnia and aggravate sinus problems.

## Sigmoid

The sigmoid bowel container at the end of the descending colon collects increasingly hardening feces if the bowels don't move regularly. As the sigmoid is a potential source of toxins affecting female reproductive organs, make sure that constipation does not occur.

## Rectum/Anus

Hemorrhoids are caused by pressure, constipation and poor bowel habits. To relieve the pain and heal the hemorrhoids, soak cotton batten in ice cold Witch Hazel liquid which has been kept in the fridge or freezer, and then insert into the anus, leaving it in for a few minutes. Repeat many times during the day, especially after bowel movements. Continue the treatment until the condition is relieved. Squatting (instead of sitting) on the toilet seat helps relieve pressure and stimulates easier, more natural bowel movments.

### NATURAL TREATMENTS FOR THE DIGESTIVE SYSTEM

*Diet*: Eat simple, light foods; eat less; avoid bran as it depletes calcium; eat nutritious seaweeds, sprouts and soups – all vegetarian, organic, alkaline foods; use the liver cleanse drink, the purification and mono diets, and juice fasts as explained in *Herbs of Grace*; avoid alcohol, fried foods, fats, non–organic minerals, eggs, meat and sugar.

*Herbs*: Dandelion, Chickweed, Fenugreek, Ginger, Gentian, Golden Seal, Marshmallow, Slippery Elm and Yellow Dock; useful herbal formulae are: Alkaline, Bowel Rejuvenator and Vitalizer, Stomach Acid/Alkaline, Exhaustion, Liver/Gall Bladder and Pancreas.

*Therapies*: Apply Castor oil packs over the abdomen and liver, and cold abdominal packs over the pancreas as needed; enemas, implants and colonics should be administered minimally and only when necessary, as it is important not to create dependence or to allow treatments to replace normal functions.

# ENDOCRINE AND REPRODUCTIVE SYSTEMS

## Adrenals

The adrenals are often exhausted and depleted by the time we reach our forties. Because many women respond to menopause with increased fear and anxiety, the adrenals are further stressed. The adrenals are considered one of the main areas for prevention, rejuvenation and support. They are also important because of the hormonal role they play during the mid–life change.

One of the main causes of reduced levels of androgen–based estrogen is stress, which depletes the adrenal glands and limits their ability to function. The main effects of adrenal malfunction are inhibition of the manufacture of twenty–eight individual hormones, decreased ability to digest foods (especially carbohydrates, sugar and minerals), lack of support for thyroid functions, reduced energy and the inability to synthesize the adrenaline and noradrenaline hormones in response to stress.

Stress depletes, exhausts and deprives the body of vitamins and minerals. According to Dr. Hans Selye, stress triggers three distinct stages or reactions: the Alarm Reaction Stage of hyperfunctioning adrenals with excess hormones; the Resistance Stage which stimulates adrenal adaptation, drawing energy and nutrients from reserves; and the Exhaustion Stage where both the body's energy and nutrition are depleted, causing chronic fatigue.

Symptoms of adrenal malfunction include fatigue, low stamina, addictions to sweet and salty foods, sensitivity to cold and low blood pressure. Adrenal symptoms can become confused with menopausal symptoms because hyperfunctioning adrenals cause high blood pressure, hot flashes, dizziness, headaches, and masculine tendencies, including face and body hair growth. Hypofunctioning adrenals can also predispose women to chronic conditions such as allergies, diabetes and hypoglycemia. Adrenal stimulation causes increased sweat gland activity which contributes to night sweats, another menopausal symptom. The continued use of stimulants and excessive exercise keeps the adrenals charged, preventing them from resting and rejuvenating.

## NATURAL TREATMENT FOR THE ADRENAL GLANDS

*Diet:* Dietary sea vegetables offer rich sources of minerals, trace minerals, protein and sodium alginate that help detoxify heavy metals from the body; eat plenty of fresh, organic vegetables, greens, legumes and fruit; chocolate cravings satisfy the need for magnesium and copper which are better supplied through diet and herbs; restore vitamin B complex depletion by the use of blackstrap molasses, yeast flakes, beans, whole grains and B complex supplements; vitamin C, zinc and manganese are essential to restore the adrenals.

*Herbs:* Rejuvenate the adrenals with the Adrenal herbal formula which contains equal parts of Borage, Mullein, Lobelia, Ginseng, Gotu Kola, Hawthorn berries and Parsley root; other useful herbal formulae are the Alkaline, Calcium, Exhaustion, Anemia and Multi/Vitamin/Mineral Naturally that replenish magnesium, calcium, zinc, potassium, sodium, copper, iodine, iron and trace minerals. Strengthen the nervous system with any of the nerve formulae, as well as the

Sweet Sleep or Lady Slipper/Valerian formulae before sleep to support and rebuild the adrenals, and assist the healing process.

Use Bach flower remedies: *Rescue Remedy* for stress; *Olive* for deep exhaustion; *Hornbeam* for fatigue with life; *Vervain* for hyperactive functioning; *Wild Rose* for apathy; *White Chestnut* for worry that repeats endlessly in the mind; *Mimulus* for anxiety; *Centaury* to increase the ability to say no and refuse domination; *Scleranthus* to make decisions; and *Mustard* for depression.

*Therapies:* Get help to release old traumas; stop overworking; take time for relaxation, leisure, and exercise; walk in nature; stop worrying; get in touch with feelings and honor them by communicating the truth; create a moderate schedule; don't waste time and energy on people and activities that aren't important; change your priorities; learn how to say no; live the grace of leisure, the elegance of moderation and the treasure of relaxation.

## Mammary Glands

The breasts are affected by stress and toxins and are connected in direct relationship to the ovaries and uterus. Toxins and pollutants are released into breast milk. Women who nurse babies knows that suckling contracts the uterus after childbirth. We also know that ovarian cycles cause our breasts to swell before periods. Breast lumps, cysts, fibroids and tumors are a result of physical, emotional and mental systemic toxicity, related closely to ovarian function. Feminine breasts have become the focus of diseases at an ever–increasing rate. They are meant to be fountains of love, comfort and nourishment but they are now retaining the disease and despair of this planet, as well as reflecting difficulties in giving and receiving love. We must change this cycle of destruction and bring the positive feminine into our lives and this world.

## Pancreas Gland

The pancreas is a glandular organ that represents the sweetness of life or the lack of it. Its ability to regulate blood sugar and energy plays a large part in avoiding fatigue from hypoglycemia and blood sugar problems, or sweet cravings that cause further imbalances and difficulties. Cravings for sugar and sweet tastes help to compensate for the lack of sweetness in our lives. There is much to explore in terms of emotional correspondences. Drink Licorice tea to stabilize the blood sugar. Take the Pancreas herbal formula. Eat natural sweet fruits and dried fruits to satisfy sweet cravings, and use honey or maple syrup for natural sweeteners.

## Parathyroid Glands

Parathyroid gland malfunction may contribute to bone loss or osteoporosis, because this gland helps to regulate the amount of calcium in the blood. If there is too much calcium in the blood it is deposited on bone and joints, causing inflammatory conditions which eventually result in arthritis. If there is not enough calcium available in the blood, it is drawn from the bones into the blood, thus depleting the bones. A high protein diet causes calcium problems due to hyperacid blood. Hyperparathyroidism causes softening of bones, destruction of bone and the development of fibrous cysts on the bone. It is essential that regular and adequate amounts of natural calcium be available during all phases of women's lives.

## Pineal Gland

As the regulator of the spiritual life and higher mind this gland affects our 'will–to–be' and our potential to evolve. It is essential to activate its positive influence through meditation, prayer and spiritual practices, so that we can be nourished by its essence. The pineal also responds to the influence of the cosmos, the stars, plants, seasons, numbers, rays, colors, vibrations, sound and light, connecting the macrocosm of universal destiny to the microcosm of our personal destiny. The more we awaken our consciousness the more we flow with our mutable evolutionary life journey. With the support of our pineal we can harmonize with the constantly changing influences of our inner and outer worlds and make our journey more conscious and more enjoyable.

Melatonin, the primary product of the pineal, is immune enhancing and sperm inhibiting in the male. It is produced almost exclusively during darkness. The eye–pineal connection is responsive to light and dark, and influences breeding cycles and birthrates whenever there are extended seasonal days and nights.

## Pituitary Gland

The pituitary plays a major role in menopause, both from the physical point of view as well as the mental and spiritual aspects of our being that are seeking to evolve so they can support our life transition toward our highest purpose. This forehead center is the home of the third eye which spiritual aspirants seek to open through prayer and meditation. This 'master' gland balances the endocrine orchestra, primarily the thyroid, adrenals and ovaries, which all contribute major influences to our mid–life change. One of the pituitary's secretions affects the absorption of calcium from nutrients in the bowels, contributing to calcium balance in the blood, and therefore bone health, a great concern during and after menopause. Skin pigmentation, another aging symptom, is stimulated by secretions from the middle lobe of the pituitary. The pituitary is also the primary producer of follicular stimulating hormones (FSH) which increase during the transition. Pituitary functions can be disturbed by stress, so it is important to this gland's function to maintain emotional equilibrium. The pituitary benefits from meditation because this focuses, calms and balances the energy at the brow center.

## Thymus Gland

This gland resides in our heart center and is affected by our ability to give and receive love. It is an important part of our immune system as well as a member of the endocrine orchestra. Malfunction of the thymus gland reduces the production of Thymosin hormones and the development of 'T' lymphocytes, which secrete a substance that attacks the protein of tumor cells, foreign cells and microorganisms. The development of chronic and degenerative conditions are liable to increase without the natural protection of thymus gland functions. If menopausal women open to cosmic levels of spirituality, increasing their abilities to give and receive unconditional love, the thymus will reflect that energy with an increased ability to protect us with its immune enhancing functions.

## Thyroid Gland

The thyroid resides in the throat center. It is the home of the ether element which strives to help us speak and hear truth, to activate our highest level of discrimination, and turn the tide of desire for the world toward longing for spiritual union with the divine. Any inhibition of this expression affects the thyroid gland which in turn affects our entire metabolism. Imbalances of any of the functions of the throat, voice box, thyroid and parathyroid glands are influenced by this elemental force. Because the thyroid gland is the conductor of the endocrine glands and is closely connected with the parasympathetic nervous system, which regulates heart, lungs and abdominal organs in response to pituitary and pineal guidance, its function greatly influences the ovaries and the adrenals, which control estrogen production.

A hypofunctioning thyroid can produce symptoms such as fatigue, low blood pressure, dizziness, poor memory and lack of concentration, which doctors may constellate under the menopause syndrome. A hyperactive thyroid stresses the adrenal glands and may cause symptoms listed above, as well as loss of body weight that decreases the body's capability to produce estrogen in body fat. Thyroid hormones are directly related to energy output, are manufactured from iodine and tyrosine and are directly responsive to the pituitary which releases thyroid stimulating hormone (TSH). Thyroid disorders affect the ovarian cycle and calcium metabolism which in turn affect the menopausal experience.

## Uterus

Because the uterus is the ark of menopause and the focus of the change, we need to recognize that its evolution into non–bleeding affects our entire feminine body and being, and our entire body and being affect it during this process. Move out of linear thinking where the uterus is considered separately, into holistic thinking where connections are acknowledged between one's life, thoughts, feelings and the condition. Visualize the inner ecology of the uterus within the pelvis, the pelvis within the body and then the body within the influences of our emotional, mental and spiritual life. Women's bodies shelter the uterus where the elements enlivened by spirit create lives which are born into the world womb. It is essential to reconnect with the sacred womb, to stay present with it through our menopausal change and to support its transition as we evolve to a higher level of cosmic creativity. The uterus is such a focus for our life experience that women create diseases out of the emotional wounds they are unable to contain within its sanctuary. Mid–life is our time to release, clear and move on. Rather than having the uterus removed, let's support its healing and keep its nurturing influence within us.

If we protect our womb throughout our life, and keep it clean, clear and free from physical and emotional toxins, we will not have to do this work during our change of life. Whenever we make a decision that affects our womb, there is a price to pay. If we make choices to use chemical douches, sprays and contraceptives, and chlorine bleached products, we must also take responsibility for their effect on our tender, sensitive and vulnerable inner tissues. Avoid tampons entirely, or change them often. Buy underwear made from natural fabrics. Consider the effect of excessive and indiscriminate sexuality. Honor and stay in touch with the inner feminine so that it will serve us in all the different dimensions of life experience.

The womb has an energetic contribution beyond its physical function in the body. It is connected to acupuncture meridians and subtle energies, far beyond the lymphatic and circulatory systems. Women who have hysterectomies never anticipate what they will feel like when their womb is gone. They never realize how it will affect their sexuality, their emotions and their energy. Women weep when they share their stories about the effect of the loss of their womb on their lives. Male doctors cannot appreciate women's relationships with their wombs.

We all know that surgery is wonderful when it saves life and relieves pain, but as women we need to learn how to live in our bodies so that we are not forced into life–and–death situations and emergency choices. It takes many years for the body to produce disease conditions, so women must learn to tune in at a much earlier stage and prevent the development of severe health problems.

## Vagina, Cervix

Women often develop abnormal vaginal conditions during menopause. The same causes that are listed in the uterus section also apply to the vagina. The labia, vagina and cervix are the entrance to the womb and they are affected by the healthy or unhealthy condition of the pelvic ecology within the entire body's inner ecology. Cervical dysplasia, or pre–cancerous changes of the tissues in the cervix, are a common problem as women age, as are discharges, unpleasant odors, warts, itching and Candida. A woman's sexual life contributes to changes in tissues, infections and discharges because we share body secretions with our sexual partners. Excessive sexual activity, especially when combined with chemical contraceptives and douches, irritate delicate female tissues. It is important to maintain moderate living habits and natural self care.

## NATURAL TREATMENT FOR THE ENDOCRINE REPRODUCTIVE SYSTEMS

Because this is so fully covered in the next section, please refer to the appropriate symptom and condition heading. Herbs, naturopathic treatments and natural living are proven and successful preventive and healing measures.

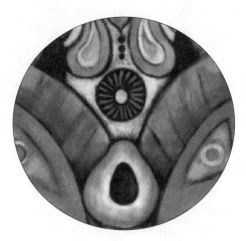

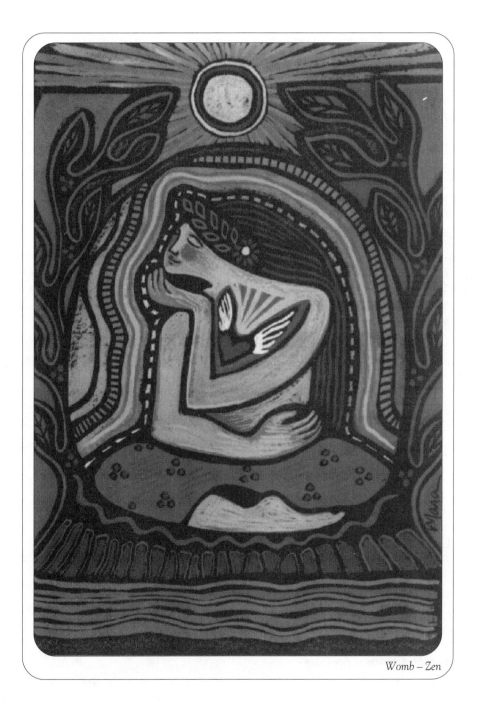

Womb – Zen

# LYMPHATIC SYSTEM

The healthy condition of our lymphatic system is essential to help us through our menopausal changes. Unfortunately many women arrive at mid–life with the lymphatic immune system already burdened by the gradual buildup of toxins and by the increasingly inadequate function of the eliminative organs. Suppression of acute conditions by the use of antibiotic drugs also contributes to the inability of our immune systems to protect us from the development of chronic conditions. A fortunate by–product of the AIDS epidemic is that it has helped the public to become more aware of the importance of the lymphatic immune system. We must learn to live healthy lives and keep our bodies clean and clear so that our natural immunity will function well.

### Adenoids

This warning device at the back of the nose is meant to protect us from infection, catarrh and mucus buildup in the nasal areas, but it becomes congested due to disordered digestion. It is out first line of defence against toxic foods. Allergies, a chronic symptom of an encumbered, underfunctioning immune system, can stress this area further. Use dietary therapy and herbs to activate and purify the lymphatic system and restore healthy function.

### Appendix

This digestive warning device in the lower ascending colon secretes antiseptic lubricant to help avoid toxic accumulation, infection and inflammation in the bowels.

### Lymph Glands

These glands are in every part of the body except the central nervous system, helping to cleanse tissues and provide immune protection. Their support is essential during menopause. They are activated by exercise, particularly to the neck, arm and groin areas. Pumping, walking or jumping movements help to stimulate the flow of lymph.

### Lacteals

Fat is absorbed into the blood in safe amounts via the lacteals in the small intestines.

### Lymph Glands – Cervicals

These neck lymph glands warn and protect us against infection in the throat and head.

### Lymph Glands – Inguinal

The lymph glands in the groin warn us and protect us against pelvic infection. This information is particularly essential during mid–life.

### Lymph Glands – Axilliary

These underarm, breast and shoulder glands warn us and protect us against toxic buildup in the breast area, so important during mid–life. Regular self massage of the breasts, underarm and shoulder areas is a valuable contribution to preventive health.

## Peyers Patches

This lymphatic area in the small intestines produces fevers to resist infections in the gastrointestinal tract.

## Thymus

The endocrine member of the lymphatic system, the thymus's protective immune functions are described in the endocrine system.

## Tonsils

This gland at the back of the throat may get sore or infected when the lymph glands cannot handle an infection. When tonsils are removed in childhood, the loss of this warning function contributes to the buildup of more chronic problems.

## Spleen

The spleen has many different functions because it reproduces the functions of all the other parts of the lymphatic system whenever this is needed. It directly affects blood purity and quality and supports liver function. When the spleen is deficient some of its activities are taken on by the bone marrow. The spleen has other subtle functions which affect our ability to receive nourishment. It also acts as a balancer of the different elements of the body. There is a close relationship between the spleen and the liver in Chinese medicine. A healthy spleen and lymphatic system are necessary for a carefree mid–life transition.

### NATURAL TREATMENT FOR THE LYMPHATIC SYSTEM

*Diet*: Avoid mucus forming and acidic foods.

*Herbs*: Use Lymphatic, Chronic, Antibiotics Naturally and the Infection herbal formulae; Echinacea, Osha root, Mullein and Lobelia are effective individually or in combination for swollen gland poultices.

*Therapies*: Lymph massage, reflexology, stimulating massage and exercise are the key therapies. Movement is the key support for lymphatic fluid which relys on muscular pumping to move it around the body. The lymphatic system does not have a pump of its own, like the heart of the circulatory system. It has one way valves which receive the lymphatic fluid and retain it, until it is moved forward and upward by the pressure of more fluid coming into the valve. Because the lymphatic system is closely associated with either retaining or releasing emotions, release of the fluids supports release of emotions and release of emotions supports release of the congested fluids. Polarity Therapy is an effective means of balancing the body and supporting release. Acupuncture is also a valuable treatment. Whenever any eliminative system is congested, activation of other systems relieves and supports its healing. Because the immune system is so burdened by this polluted modern world, we must make every effort possible to maintain and preserve its functions.

# MUSCULAR SYSTEM

The quality of our body tissues, ligaments and muscles depends on the ability of our blood and circulation to nourish us, on the lymphatic system to purify body fluids and tissues, on the digestive system to provide nutrients, and on the respiratory system to bring oxygen to the cells. Chemistry imbalances, toxic overloads, lack of exercise, increasing acidity, stress, a sedentary lifestyle, anxiety and constipation all collaborate to increase toxins in our body tissues.

Women often sacrifice their health, personal time and exercise to fulfill work, family and social duties and responsibilities. Although there is a great emphasis now on keeping fit and working out, many women are not able to fit exercise into their busy lives. Magazines and television continually present us with visions of material and physical perfection. We clean and wash and iron and dress, work night and day, shop, play hard, and live life on the run. Menopause is the time to prune, pare down, trim and simplify. We must look at our lives and find a way to reduce unnecessary activities so that we can find time to exercise and live a quality lifestyle which is balanced in all realms of activity.

Women complain of cellulite, weakness, excess weight, water retention, as well as aches, pains and soreness that eventually develop into chronic conditions in the muscles, tissues, joints and tendons. Movement is life. Blood and lymph must flow in order to nourish and cleanse our cells and tissues. Toxins must be removed on a daily basis. Life and energy must flow through every cell and tissue if we are to remain well. If we don't find the time to do this, eventually the time will be taken from us through illness.

## NATURAL TREATMENT FOR THE MUSCULAR SYSTEM

*Diet:* Eat alkaline, vegetarian foods, and include seaweeds on a daily basis; eat the purification diet for a week or two, twice yearly, eat mono meals, one food per meal, whenever possible.

*Herbs:* The Body Building, Alkaline, Multi/Mineral/Vitamin Naturally, Calcium, Arthritis and Anti–Inflammatory herbal formulae can be used as required; Alfalfa is an excellent natural supplement because of its high content of natural trace minerals.

*Therapies:* Movement is necessary to keep the muscles alive, clean and well; stretch, dance, swim, walk and practice yoga or tai chi; keep life moving.

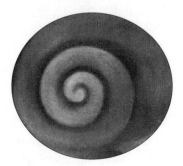

# NERVOUS SYSTEM

Our nervous system must be alive and strong to help us through our mid–life years. Adrenal exhaustion, stress, anxiety, overwork, poor diet, lack of leisure and exercise, shocks, accidents, in short, life itself, all take their toll on the nervous system. The nervous system must be nourished and replenished on a daily basis. In modern life many of us are sympathetic nervous system dominant, or yang and active, as we constantly deal with the stresses of daily life and the outward direction of the world. However, we must develop and activate the yin and inactive parasympathetic nervous system to help us relax, enable us to enjoy quiet and leisure and assist us to rest and rejuvenate.

Because our nervous system is our communicating system we rely on its strength to keep our body, mind and emotions working together. If we are over sensitive our sympathetic nervous system is exhausted and we have to use our energy to protect ourselves, or we may have to draw away from full participation in life.

Strong emotions and fears deplete the nervous system. Fear keeps us in a constant state of anxiety that will not allow us to sleep deeply or to turn off our 'fight and flight' adrenal readiness. Anger, jealousy, rage and bitterness acidify our body and upset the ability of the nervous system to function adequately. Mental and emotional illness draws away the reserves of the nervous system. Dependence on tranquilizers, sedatives and sleeping pills dull the communicating aspect of the nervous system and separate us from the truth of our problems.

## NATURAL TREATMENT FOR THE NERVOUS SYSTEM

*Diet*: Avoid caffeine, sugar, chocolate, alcohol, meat, and chemical preservatives and dyes; do not stimulate the body for short term energy; take regular high calcium foods; a vegetarian diet of wholesome natural foods is highly recommended, as excess protein diets and junk foods deplete calcium from the system.

*Herbs*: Take the Adrenal, Calcium, Nerve Rejuvenator, Nerve Vitalizer, Nerve Tonic and Adrenal formulae; drink calming herbs such as Horsetail, Catnip, Chamomile, Vervain and Valerian before sleep; Bach flower and homeopathic remedies are very useful to clear mental and emotional disturbances that weaken the nervous system, however, the nervous system must also be nourished and strengthened through nutrients available in quality foods and herbs.

*Therapies*: Live a lifestyle that is not based on stress and overwork; make sure you get adequate sleep and even indulge in occasional naps; take rejuvenating holidays; learn to relax, slow down, and enjoy the present; enjoy quality leisure; learn to be a human 'be–ing,' not just a human 'do–ing'; release old traumas locked in the body; polarity therapy offers sympathic nervous system balancing and parasympathetic activation; enjoy regular relaxing aromatherapy and Epsom salts baths; study and practice yoga, tai chi, meditation, relaxation techniques and stress release exercises to learn how to activate the parasympathetic nervous system; walk regularly in natural surroundings; release static electricity by walking barefoot in the home and on the ground; aerobic exercises will release stress and allow deeper levels of relaxation.

# SKELETAL SYSTEM

Our skeletal system is our support system. It gives us form and allows us to move that form. If menopausal women are stiff and rigid in structure they will find it hard to move, change, adjust and transform. The skeletal system is a reflection of our earth element and relates to the emotion of fear. We hold on because we fear the unknown. Remember the softness and flexibility of youth and keep that quality alive. Bone is alive and responds to nutrients, to movement and to life energies.

Osteoporosis and degeneration of the teeth are a potential reality for menopausal women who suffer from calcium depletion. Women's nails also reflect this condition through breakage, ridges and marks. Diseases such as arthritis and rheumatism affect movement and cause debilitating weakness especially in the knees, hips and fingers. Some women experience spinal malformations, stiffness, pain, weakness and swelling. These conditions have developed over the years through poor living habits, stress, lack of essential nutrients, disordered digestion, lack of exercise and emotional and mental distress. It's never too late to begin healing. Start now.

## NATURAL TREATMENT FOR THE SKELETAL SYSTEM

*Diet:* Include adequate organic grains, seaweeds, vegetables, nuts and seeds in daily meals.

*Herbs*: Use the Body Building, Calcium and Multi/Mineral/Vitamin herbal formulae; take Alfalfa supplements to provide trace minerals.

*Therapies*: Rolfing and deep tissue massage releases muscles from the bone, increases flexibility, and improves posture; receive regular treatments from osteopaths, cranial sacral practitioners, polarity therapists or chiropractors; study yoga, tai chi and dance; exercise and stretch regularly because lack of exercise increases bone degeneration; we get shorter as we age, so hang upside down to stretch out and release vertebrae; lie on a slant board or sleep with the feet higher than the head; practice Polarity Therapy squatting exercises; keep bending and moving; don't solidify like the pillar of salt; make flexibility a lifestyle; avoid high heel shoes which increase muscular rigidity in the legs and pelvis.

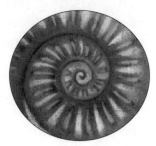

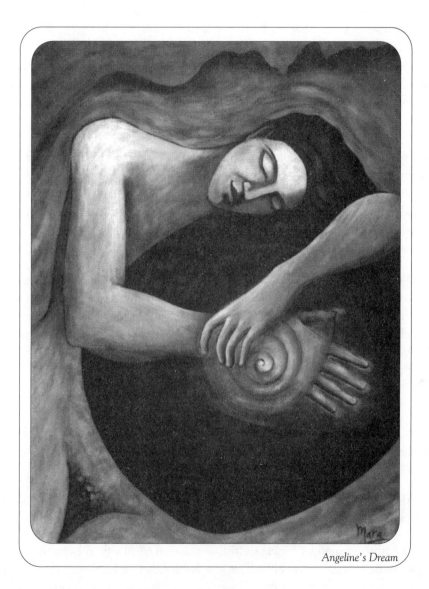

*Angeline's Dream*

# URINARY SYSTEM

Urinary conditions often accompany women's reproductive diseases and menopausal and aging processes. Infections, toxins and inflammation spread quickly through the pelvis because all the organs are touching one other, and the blood and lymph flow through all the tissues. Women may complain of lower back ache that is actually caused by kidney problems. Listen to the body and learn to heed symptoms at an early stage. Don't put off dealing with pain or malfunction, no matter how busy work and life may be. Search out and create a support system. Study natural health. Create a home library of reference books. Keep a collection of herbs to use whenever acute conditions occur. Study and apply the information in *Herbs of Grace*.

## Bladder

Bladder troubles accompany mid–life and aging due to increased acidity and sensitivity. Leakage, incontinence, or excessive night urination may also become a problem. Infections may occur; the many causes include drug reactions, childbirth difficulties, accidents, surgery after–effects, alcohol use, constipation, fibroids and cysts, and the thinning of the bladder wall during menopause.

## Kidneys

The seat of essential energy or *chi* according to the Chinese, the kidneys are important to the aging and menopause process. They are our bottom line organ because they try to accomplish whatever is left undone by other eliminative organs and systems. They strive to balance acid and alkaline, and eliminate through the urine whatever is needed to be released to keep that balance. Support the kidneys by drinking enough water and herbal teas, but not too much so that they become waterlogged.

## NATURAL TREATMENT FOR THE URINARY SYSTEM

*Diet*: Avoid colas, coffee, acid foods, citrus, tomatoes, hot spices and foods, iced or cold foods and drinks, and tobacco; drink purified or distilled water, barley water or herbal teas regularly, and cranberry juice whenever there is any infection or burning.

*Herbs:* Take the Kidney Bladder formula; Uva Ursi, Buchu, Cleavers, Parsley, Cornsilk and Marshmallow are useful individual herbs; drink Waterbalance herbal tea for prevention.

*Therapies*: Sitz baths are useful to increase the circulation of blood and lymph, to stimulate healing and to strengthen the pelvic organs; sit in a shallow bath or bowl with the legs and upper body out of the water; keep warm; sit in cold water for one minute, then in very warm water for three minutes; repeat two or three times; complete the treatment with cold; dress in cotton pajamas and walk for fifteen minutes, inside or outside, depending on energy and the weather; take acupuncture treatments; use progesterone salves made from Wild Yam root on the outer bladder tissues; use the Ginger kidney poultice as described in *Herbs of Grace*.

# SYMPTOMS & CONDITIONS

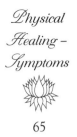

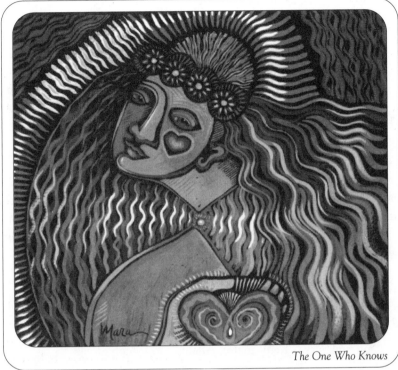

*The One Who Knows*

### ACHING JOINTS & MUSCLES

Hormone changes and calcium imbalances in the blood and bones, combined with increasing levels of acidity and toxicity, begin the chemical changes within the body that eventually produce inflammatory disease. Osteoarthritis is a condition which produces stiff, achy, lumpy, swollen, hot and cracking joints. Rheumatoid arthritis is an auto–immune disorder of swollen, tender areas combined with fever and fatigue.

*Diet:* Eat at least 80% alkaline food; take Flax seed and Evening Primrose oils as regular supplements; eliminate tomatoes, peppers, sugar, potatoes, eggplant, citrus, meat, vegetable oils and MSG; drink adequate water and fresh vegetable juice; eat seaweeds regularly.

*Herbs:* Use the Arthritis and the Anti–Inflammatory formulae; natural aspirin salicylates are abundant in the bark, buds and leaves of the Birches, Willows and Poplars, as well as in Black Haw, Wintergreen and Black Currant buds; steroid rich herbs that ease sore joints are Black Cohosh, Devil's Claw or Club, Ginseng, Poke root, Sarsaparilla and Wild Yam.

*Homeopathy:* *Arbutus Andrachne* for gouty, rheumatic, arthritic symptoms, especially in the larger joints; *Bryonia* for irritable, thirsty, apathetic types who suffer from red, swollen, hot joints; *Elaterium* for arthritic nodules; *Sulfur* for rheumatic pain, gout combined with itching on the left shoulder, sweaty hands and red lips and face.

*Therapies:* Acupuncture; Ginger kidney poultices; apply melted paraffin wax wherever there is pain or swelling; saunas, steams, mud baths, hot mineral springs and sweat lodges will release acids and ease the symptoms; keep moving, flexible, swaying, flowing, bending, circulating, softening, sweetening, loosening, stretching and reaching, swimming, yoga, tai chi and walking are helpful to keep the blood and lymph moving.

## ALLERGIES

Allergies can increase during aging and menopause as the body slows down due to increased toxicity and malfunction. Escalating stress, worry, insomnia and periodic difficulties, together with mental and emotional suffering, divorce, children leaving home, etc., all combine to increase immune insufficiency and allergic reactions.

*Diet:* Avoid mucus–forming and acidic foods as well as all foods and drinks that contain preservatives, chemicals, dyes and sugar. Dietary changes are essential and the purification, mono, alkaline, vegetarian and juice diets are most effective to reduce allergies.

*Herbs:* Take the Adrenal, Nerve Rejuvenator, Allergy and Lymph formulae.

*Homeopathy:* *Sabadilla* is useful for hay fever.

*Therapies:* Apply the full purification, regeneration and transformation regimens from three to six months for best results; take lymph massages; exercise regularly.

## BLADDER INCONTINENCE & INFECTIONS

Bladder incontinence and infections may occur during the aging and menopausal process when the system is weaker due to increased stress, acidity and toxins. The main causes (other than systemic constitutional weakness and kidney/bladder disease) are pelvic toxicity and acid/alkaline imbalance. Symptoms are varied and may be any one or more of the following: infection, burning, incontinence, aching kidneys, backache, strong urine odor, dark urine color, frequency, pain and having to get up often to pass water at night.

*Diet:* Drink barley water (wash then soak the barley overnight in water, strain off the barley water); avoid alcohol, acid foods and hot spices.

*Herbs:* Drink Waterbalance tea copiously and take acute doses of the Kidney/Bladder formula until the condition clears; Buchu and Uva Ursi are the best herbs to take on their own.

*Homeopathy:* Use *Aconitum* for scanty, red, hot, painful urine; *Terebinthina* for scanty, suppressed, bloody urine and acute inflamed kidneys.

*Therapies:* Take warm sitz baths in water or Chamomile tea; apply Ginger poultices over the kidneys at night, and massage Lavender aromatherapy oil over the bladder area in the lower pelvis and the kidneys in the lower back; take Lavender internally by mixing one drop of the oil in three ounces of water.

## BLEEDING & FLOODING – DYSMENORRHEA

Flooding has many potential causes, some of which might be cysts, fibroids, IUD's, cancer or endometriosis. Such severe symptoms almost always have emotional roots, such as marital or sexual abuse, incest and emotional and mental disorders. Ask why the womb is draining out the life's blood? What wounds are being carried and contained in the womb? Seek ways to heal the emotional roots of the condition before a hysterectomy becomes necessary.

*Diet:* Eat high iron foods such as molasses, raisins, currants, oatmeal, potatoes, greens, brown rice, seaweeds, whole wheat, and red, orange and yellow vegetables.

*Herbs:* Use the Women's Reproductive and Anemia formulae; high iron herbs will help to compensate for blood loss and give strength and energy; these are Nettles, Burdock, Chickweed, Milk Thistle, Echinacia, Fenugreek, Sarsaparilla, Yellow Dock and Dandelion; to stop or control heavy flow, drink Lady's Mantle herb tea and take high doses of Cayenne powder; use progesterone herbs to help balance hormones – refer to the appendices.

*Homeopathy:* Use *Lachesis* for dark, thick, strong blood accompanied by pain and rage; *Sepia* for draining, heavy, painful, frequent bleeding with backache, constipation and depression; *China* for exhaustion from heavy flooding with clots; *Sabina* for violent flooding with clots, cramping and weakness, which worsens with movement; *Secale* for flooding with cramps; *Sulfur* for flooding with sweats and hot flashes; *Belladonna* for bright red flooding with clots, headaches and sensitivity.

*Therapies:* Explore the emotional causes through body–centered psychotherapies such as rosenwork, polarity therapy and hakomi. Take total rest during the flooding time. Make sure the bowels are clear and avoid constipation during any part of the monthly cycle.

## BLOATING & GAS

Bloating and gas often increase during mid–life due to insufficient digestion, stress and poor chewing and eating habits. Poor digestion affects the entire system and must be corrected.

*Diet:* Eat simple combinations of alkaline food, and only allow yourself less than 20% acid foods; refer to the acid/alkaline chart in *Herbs of Grace*; avoid combining proteins and fruits, and proteins and starches; eat fruit alone, especially melons; eat proteins alone at the beginning of the meal; go on a mono diet or a juice fast to give the digestive system a rest, and then pay attention when you bring back individual foods, so that you can determine which ones are causing the problems; chew slowly and eat in a relaxed manner; do not drink with meals or drink very hot or very cold liquids, as this slows down digestion.

*Herbs:* Individual herbs such as Dong Quai and Wild Yam root are useful to reduce bloating and gas; take the Stomach Acid/Alkaline and the Bowel Rejuvenator formulae regularly over several months; other herbs which relieve gas are Catnip, Ginger, Fennel, Garlic, Papaya, Peppermint, Spearmint and Thyme.

*Homeopathy: Bryonia, Chamomilla, Chelidonium, Gentian, Lycopodium, Nux Vomica* and *Pulsatilla* are suggested; consult a practitioner or read a homeopathic guide to determine which is the correct remedy.

*Therapies:* Chew food well; apply a cold abdominal pack for one half hour when there is bloating; clear any constipation and make sure the bowels are moving at least twice a day.

## BLOOD FLOW ABSENCE – AMENORRHEA

Absence of blood flow during menopause may be normal. Cessation of menses due to emotional stress, starvation, excessive exercise or dieting, and disordered digestive habits is considered a health problem.

*Diet:* Evening Primrose oil and vitamin E are useful when taken internally; strive for moderation in eating, drinking and make efforts to establish moderate living habits.

*Herbs:* Drink Nettle, Dong Quai or Pennyroyal tea for three days during the new moon to help this condition, and take the Hormone and Female Reproductive formulae; take bowel rejuvenating herbs to relieve the system.

*Homeopathy: Pulsatilla* for suppressed and tardy menses from nervous debility, often accompanied by fatigue and back pain; *Graphites* for late menstruation with constipation, pale, thin leucorrhoea and swollen, hard breasts; *Natrum Muriaticum* for suppressed and irregular menses, when there is a dry vagina, and watery, acrid leucorrhoea.

*Therapies:* Try psychotherapy, counseling and bodywork, together with Castor oil packs as described in *Herbs of Grace*, to relax pelvic tension, soften impacted feces, and release blockages in the pelvis that affect cyclic blood flow and hormonal balance.

## BLOOD SPOTTING

Hormonal changes and imbalances are often the causes of spotting. A medical exam will confirm that it isn't caused by cancer, hyperplasia, polyps, cervical dysplasia, miscarriage or fibroids.

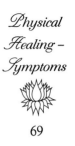
*Diet:* Eat high iron alkaline foods.

*Herbs:* Drink two cups of Red Raspberry leaf tea, and one cup of Ginger root tea daily; use Cinnamon on food and in tea; Cinnamon also stops diarrhea; to prevent mid–cycle blood spotting increase progesterone precursors by using Chasteberry, Sarsaparilla, Wild Yam or Yarrow herb; Lady's Mantle and False Unicorn are also useful to stop spotting.

*Homeopathy:* Use *China* if spotting is combined with weakness and depression, and *Pulsatilla* when strong emotions are combined with the bleeding.

*Therapies:* Keep the bowels clean and clear; avoid using tampons; rest and relax during periods; massage the female reproductive reflex areas around the ankles on the feet .

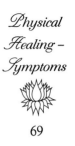

## BREAST LUMPS, CYSTS, TUMORS & CANCER

The breasts gather congestion and toxicity due to emotions, life stresses, systemic depletion and malfunction, and also in relation to what is happening in the bowels, the ovaries and uterus. When I created breast cancer in my twenties, I did not know then that it was related to bowel toxins in my ascending colon – the relationship can be observed in my iris. A three–month purification program as described in the Healing Grace chapter in *Herbs of Grace* cleared this condition and I have been completely free of any reoccurrence for the last twenty five years.

*Diet:* Include mono, alkaline, vegetarian, organic, wholefood, and purifying foods in the daily diet, take fresh juices regularly, eat seaweeds and make the potassium broth.

*Herbs:* Blood Purifying, Liver/Gall Bladder, Bowel Rejuvenator, Bowel Vitalizer, Lymphatic, Chronic Purifier, Circulation and Antibiotics Naturally formulae; drink four cups a day of Red Clover and Red Raspberry tea; great success stories have been told about the Essiac herbal cancer formula which is composed of Burdock root, Slippery Elm, Sheep Sorrel and Turkey Rhubarb; take high amounts of thyroid and liver herbs, especially Milk Thistle, together with therapeutic doses of potassium from Elderflower.

*Homeopathy: Iodum* for thin, dark complexioned women with a strong appetite, who have a tendency towards enlarged lymphatic glands, dwindling mammary glands and nodosities on the breasts.

*Treatments:* Take lymph massage, press reflexology points on the feet, and massage the breasts regularly; apply Castor oil packs over the liver, abdomen and breast areas, and herbal Poke root poultices on the breast; Chaparral baths are also useful to aid detoxification; the earlier natural treatments are applied, the better; consider a visit to the Gerson Cancer Clinic.

## BREAST SENSITIVITY & SWELLING

Hormone imbalances and cyclic changes may result in swollen and sore breasts, especially during the estrogen cycles which lead up to the monthly flow. As the uterus fills with blood, the breasts also become enlarged, engorged and sensitive.

*Diet:* Avoid coffee, colas, and black tea because caffeine increases breast swelling, tenderness and lumps; take high doses of vitamin E and natural calcium regularly; take foods high in calcium, magnesium and vitamin B.

*Herbs:* Black Cohosh, Chasteberry, Dong Quai, and Liferoot relieve this condition; apply poultices of cabbage leaves, or Lobelia and Mullein; massage the breasts regularly with St. Joan's Wort oil.

*Homeopathy:* Use *Sanguinaria* for breast soreness when symptoms are stronger on the right side of the body and when there is burning during offensive, profuse menses; *Arnica* for sore nipples; *Chamomilla* when the nipples are inflamed and tender to the touch and there is peevish restlessness, sensitivity, irritability and snappish impatience.

*Therapies:* Massage the breasts thoroughly around ovulation to increase the flow of lymph and energy; apply the Castor oil pack on the breasts and abdomen three nights in a row during the first week after ovulation.

## CANDIDA, THRUSH, & YEAST INFECTIONS

Candida and other yeast infections are a sign that changes in body chemistry and tissues are burdening the immune system, and that the condition has gone beyond the body's ability to eliminate and clear the infection. These conditions involve the entire gastrointestinal tract and can extend into other body orifices as well. Symptoms can include fatigue, sweet cravings, irritability, vaginal itching, discharges, odor and frequent infections.

Deep purification, regeneration and balancing of the entire body system is essential. There are many books written on the natural and orthodox healing of Candida and Thrush, but symptomatic efforts are not enough. The lymphatic and immune system must be relieved by direct activation. The activity of all the eliminative channels and the liver must be increased.

*Diet:* Strict dietary reform is necessary; avoid fruit, grain, yeast bread, brewer's yeast, cultured cheeses, alcohol, and sugar; use Garlic, olive oil and Cayenne on food instead of complicated dressings and seasonings. Pay attention to dietary combinations. The mono diet is best and will give the quickest improvement. Sometimes fruit can be eaten alone on an empty stomach.

*Herbs:* Take Echinacea and other immune stimulants internally; clear constipation; use the herbal Yellow Dock douche regularly with the vaginal ovule; take the Fungus formula internally as well as an individual systemic herbal nutrient mix prescribed by a natural health practitioner; effective douches are Golden Seal, Garlic, apple cider vinegar, yogurt, acidophilus and wheatgrass; Pau D'Arco and Black Walnut are also antifungal; make a douche of Rose, Lavender and Bergamot aromatherapy oils, in one pint of warm water, then shake well and douche.

*Homeopathy:* Use individual remedies for specific symptoms and personality type.

*Therapies:* Use douches and enemas as required, and administer a course of the vaginal ovule treatment as outlined in *Herbs of Grace;* avoid spermicides, vaginal contraceptive creams, chemical douches and sprays, and synthetic underwear and pantyhose.

## CERVICAL DYSPLASIA

Cervical cancer is on the increase due to the increase of unnatural living and an increasingly polluted environment. Chemical contraception methods, synthetic hormones, spermicides, douches, disordered diet, and immoderate living habits combined with sexual excesses and promiscuity have lead to a breakdown in systemic functions. Addictions to alcohol, cigarettes and drugs, together with the negative influences from computers, television, processed foods and drinks, chemicals and dyes, also contribute to disordered body functions and weaker immune systems. The ark of life, the female reproductive system is becoming diseased at ever–increasing rates, even in young women. The internal feminine environment is mirroring our dysfunctional modern world. Both the inner and outer ecologies are suffering.

When the cervix begins to form abnormal cells, orthodox medicine offers laser surgery and other drastic means, yet it does not deal with the causes in the life of the woman. I have worked with many women who were able to completely reverse this condition with natural treatment. When clients make efforts to achieve lifestyle changes and follow through with a six–month purification, regeneration and transformation program, results can be completely successful. In some cases a medical doctor referred the clients to me, and the improvements were documented before and after with medical tests, demonstrating complete recovery.

*Diet:* Alkaline, vegetarian, purifying and mono diets, and fresh juices are recommended.

*Herbs:* The complete inner ecology herbal nutrient program must be administered, and should include the Female Reproductive, Bowel, Chronic Purifying and Lymphatic formulae; administer the vaginal ovule and douche herbal treatment over several weeks.

*Homeopathy:* Use *Carbo Animalis* for older patients who are sad, reflective, quiet and who wish to be alone; *Iodum* when there is uterine hemorrhage or pain from the ovary to uterus along with acrid leucorrhoea; *Kreosotum* for peevish childlike personalities who are suffering from cancerous conditions accompanied by itching in the vulva, labia and vagina; *Thuja* when the vagina is sensitive, and warts, leucorrhoea and pain are present.

*Therapies:* Use herbal and aromatherapy alternately hot and cold sitz baths, douches and herbal vaginal steams, together with counseling and flower essences for the emotional imbalances.

## CONCENTRATION, MEMORY PROBLEMS & DIZZINESS

Forgetfulness, lack of concentration, poor memory, dizziness and fuzzy-headedness are also symptoms which cause menopausal women suffering. Aside from circulatory, toxic and hormonal causes, this state can also be a positive sign of returning to right brain intuitive thought processes. Instead of fighting and fearing this change, sink into it and allow answers to come in a new way. Take into consideration the Circulatory Hardening constitutional type in the *Herbs of Grace* Iricology chapter, and study and apply the recommendations.

*Diet:* Avoid eggs, oils, fats, salt, alcohol, and fried foods; take lecithin daily to help reduce cholesterol levels; avoid the intake of minerals by drinking only distilled water; do not use any inorganic supplements or aspirin.

*Herbs:* Use the Circulation Systemic and Cerebral formulae, as well as Ginkgo and Gotu Kola; drink Buckwheat tea; the Liver and Lymphatic herbal formulae are also essential to help clean the blood before it returns to the circulatory system.

*Homeopathy:* There are so many remedies listed under the 'Mind' section in the homeopathic Materia Medica, it is necessary to have a consultation to determine the appropriate remedy.

*Therapies:* Exercise daily; sleep with the head down and the feet raised; practice yoga inversion postures.

## CRAMPING

Cramping reveals the tension in the pelvis and the pain speaks what is not being spoken. Women accumulate and contain emotional suffering in their womb. Cramping is also caused by calcium deficiency, by endometrisis, by toxic and inflammatory pelvic conditions, by constipation and by pressure from other organs. Spinal misalignment and poor posture will also contribute to cramping. Much improvement can be accomplished by taking time off during the monthly flow to lie still, take the attention into the womb and practice visualization to release tension. Pelvic exercise will increase energy and circulation to the area. Rolfing and deep tissue massage will also stimulate release. Dietary, herbal and therapeutic supports are superb supports to any program. It is important to approach healing from different points of view and find what works.

*Diet:* Eat lightly immediately before and during the menses; take high calcium foods regularly.

*Herbs:* Take the Period Pain formula from the onset of the period; take the Women's Reproductive and the Calcium formulae throughout the month; Black Haw and Cramp bark reduce cramping and flooding with their powerful astringent antispasmodic actions, as well as containing hormonal precursors; Garden Sage reduces cramps without increasing flooding; Ginger or Motherwort reduce cramps, but do not take these herbs if there is any danger of flooding; use Valerian or White Willow to reduce pain, because aspirin can increase flooding.

*Homeopathy: Secale* for severe cramps with flooding and no clots; *Sabina* for severe cramps with clots and weakness; *Chamomilla* for cramping that is relieved by heat, and accompanied by distress and irritability.

*Therapies:* Use hot water bottles on the back; practice deep relaxation, rest and breathe deeply into the pelvis; massage the reflexology points on the feet for the lower back and the uterus; press a spoon on the very back of the tongue (almost causing gagging) several times to reduce cramping; have a medical exam to make sure this is not an endometrial condition.

## CRAMPING & NUMBNESS IN THE ARMS & LEGS

Caused by lack of exercise, shortage of calcium, anemia and overuse of tobacco, cramping in the extremities can be easily remedied with natural means. Heart problems, osteoporosis and hypothyroidism could also be causal factors. Read the information on the muscular and skeletal body systems, and the osteoporosis treatment section. Avoid antidepressants and foods that deplete calcium (refer to page 144).

*Diet:* Eat calcium rich foods such as sesame seeds, seaweeds, kale, turnip, almonds and soybeans regularly; also take vitamin E; this condition could be brought on by either an overdose or a depletion of vitamin B 6.

*Herbs:* Take the Calcium formula and calcium–rich herbs such as Nettles and Horsetail; Black Haw, St. Joan's Wort and high iron Yellow Dock are also useful; drink Valerian tea before sleep.

*Homeopathy: Aconite* for numbness in the extremities especially when accompanied by fear and anxiety.

*Therapies:* Hot footbaths or baths before bed followed by a cool shower will help to relieve the cramping. Massage, deep tissue bodywork, rolfing, polarity therapy and reflexology will help to relieve this condition.

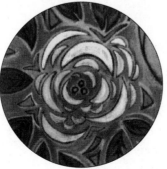

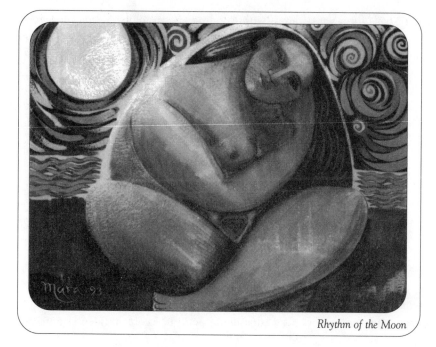

*Rhythm of the Moon*

## CYCLE INTERVALS & IRREGULARITIES

Cycle intervals and irregularities are a natural aspect of menopause, not an illness. Balance the hormones, establish a harmonious relationship with the moon, drink herbal teas, eat a moderate and healthy diet, and surrender to the change.

*Diet:* Reduce animal fats which are converted into estrogens and which may also contain injected hormones; avoid drinking recycled tap water because it may contain hormones. Sprinkle Cinnamon on food; eat foods high in bioflavinoids – wheat germ oil, vitamin E (400 to 600 I.U. daily), as well as whole grains, dark leafy green vegetables and raw nuts. Caution: take only 50 to 150 I.U. of vitamin E if there is any tendency to high blood pressure, diabetes or heart problems; avoid using birth control pills to control the menstrual cycle during menopause.

*Herbs:* Chasteberry, Cinnamon, Dong Quai, Liferoot blossoms and Red Raspberry leaves are all useful for this condition; drink a cup of Pennyroyal tea during the full moon days; use estrogen herbs and formulae.

*Homeopathy:* Use *Ambra* when the cycle is too early; *Coccus* when menses are too early or intermittent, when the flow is only in the evening and night, when profuse and black with dark clots; *Nux vomica* when menses are irregular, too early and last too long; *Phosphorus* when menses are too early, scanty and last too long; *Pulsatilla* for suppressed, late, intermittent, clotted, changeable menses; *Sepia* when menses are too late and scanty, or early and profuse when accompanied by a bearing down sensation; and *Sulfur* for late, short, scanty, difficult menses with soreness, itching and burning.

*Therapies:* Let the full moon shine through the window at night or leave on a night light during the three full moon days; become close to or live with women who are cycling with the moon and synchronize with their rhythms; watch the moon change through the month; observe the tide's ebb and flow; try acupuncture, rolfing, cranial sacral treatments, deep tissue massage to release muscles in the lower back and pelvis, and polarity therapy deep perineal and psoas release to help balance the water element and its cyclical rhythmns; exercise the pelvis and sacral areas.

## DIGESTIVE PROBLEMS

### Liver

Because part of the liver's work is to break down hormones and make their ingredients available for hormone production, this function increases during the menopause, making the liver less available for digestive processes. Constant eating also diminishes its function.

*Diet:* Avoid fats, fried foods, alcohol and eggs.

*Herbs:* Support the liver with the Liver/Gall Bladder and the Blood Purifying formulae; use Castor oil packs over the liver; use Milk Thistle and Gentian herbs to help detoxify the liver.

### Stomach

The results of years of eating and drinking disorders, junk foods, addictions, cravings and indulgences take their toll during mid–life years. It is a time to eat natural organic whole foods, become vegetarian, try juice fasts, take nourishment rich rich herbal nutrients and develop loving nurturing habits to prepare for healthy, happy, productive elder years.

Diet: Eat regularly; use simple food combinations; try the mono diet; eat seaweeds regularly; avoid acid foods and caffeine stimulants; make sure the diet is at least 80% alkaline.

*Herbs:* Drink one teaspoon Slippery Elm powder blended in one cup of warm honey water three times a day; take three to four capsules of Slippery Elm powder with each meal or mix it with food – it is excellent in cereals; use the Stomach Acid/Alkaline Balancing and Alkaline formulae, as well as Wild Yam root, Psyllium, Calamus or Gotu Kola herbs.

### Bowels

As estrogen levels decrease, the bowels slow down. The liver becomes stressed because it has to work much harder during menopause, which also contributes to constipation. Take the time to make sure the bowels move regularly every day; use herbal laxatives and any of the bowel formulae; take enemas when necessary; avoid antibiotics that will reduce bowel function.

*Diet:* Drink a full glass of lemon water on waking; add Slippery Elm to oatmeal at breakfast; drink prune juice in the morning; make sure there is enough dietary fiber, liquids, watery fruits, and vegetables; take acidophilus; avoid bran because it reduces calcium levels and encourages bone loss, and inorganic iron supplements, which create constipation; take the iron rich herb, Yellow Dock, or Ferr. Phos. tissue salts.

*Herbs:* The herbal Enema Mix formula of Burdock, Yellow Dock, Red Raspberry and Red Clover stimulates the liver to dump bile and increase bowel action and cleansing; use Calamus, Alfalfa, Dandelion and Yellow Dock herbs, either the Bowel Vitalizer or Bowel Rejuvenator formulae, Slippery Elm drinks, seaweeds, and Psyllium or Flax seeds to keep the bowels moving.

## DISCHARGES

Excessive, strong, colored or painful discharges from the vagina are evidence of functional imbalances in the reproductive organs, disturbance of the normal flow of the pelvic circulatory and lymphatic fluids, low–grade infection, tissue toxicity and inflammation. This symptom is also often related to constipation and to tense, hard pelvic muscles and tissues. Emotional holding of indiscrimate sex, repressed memories of incest, rape, violence, sexual fears, inhibitions, shame, guilt and denial also play their part in vaginal distress. Discharges may be indicative of tumors, cysts and fibroids, the physical crystallization of long–term mental and emotional distress focused within the female reproductive organs. Medical diagnosis is important to determine what is going on. It is important to apply the full internal systemic constitutional, eliminative purification, regeneration and transformation treatments as well as more specific treatments.

*Diet:* Wholefood vegetarian purification diet and juice cleanses are recommended; the mono diet is useful to determine which foods aggravate the condition.

*Herbs:* Bowel Vitalizer or Rejuvenator, Women's Reproductive, Vaginal Ovule, Circulation, Lymph and the Chronic formulae, together with a systemic constitutional herbal program.

*Homeopathy:* Because there are many types of discharges and many different homeopathic remedies for vaginal discharges, it is best to consult a homeopathic practitioner.

*Therapies:* Use herbal sitz baths; apply Chickweed, Calendula or Balm of Gilead ointments locally; use Yellow Dock vaginal douches; administer the vaginal ovule treatment as required; use yogurt or acidophilus douches to balance the vaginal bacterial climate.

## ENDOMETRIOSIS

Endometriosis develops from uterine tissue spreading and growing beyond the walls of the uterus. This abnormal condition within the uterus, occurs when endometrial tissue, normally expelled through menstruation, travels inside the body and implants itself on the fallopian tubes, ovaries, outer wall of the uterus, pelvic lining, cervix or vagina. Endometrial tissues have also been found in the intestines, appendix, rectum and even farther away. These endometrial cells eventually form patches and scars that respond monthly to estrogen menstrual hormones by enlarging, thickening and bleeding, causing severe pain. While this condition most often begins before mid–life, it progresses along with and increases difficulties with any other menopausal symptoms. Contributing to infertility, predisposition to endometriosis also occurs because of long periods of ovulation without interruption by pregnancy and lactation.

The main symptoms of endometriosis are pain and excessive bleeding, which occur most often during the monthly blood flow, but which can also be activated by urination and lovemaking. Although the above symptoms make us suspect that we have this condition, it can only be confirmed by a laparoscopy. Medical doctors usually prescribe birth control pills or advise women to consider getting pregnant, as that has been known to help shrink the endometrial tissue that is outside the womb. Various drugs have been administered, all with considerable side effects. A hysterectomy is often recommended by medical doctors, or a less extreme surgery that vaporizes endometrial tissue with a laser.

Let us consider some of the other causes of this painful and debilitating condition, such as pressure and tension in the pelvic cavity due to emotional stress, depression, anxiety and constipation. We may ask ourselves why we are bleeding inside ourselves? What pain is being experienced in the physical body that is being translated from the emotional and mental aspects of our being?

I have had personal experience with endometriosis because I created it due to severe emotional stress and shock during my divorce from my English husband. Month by month as I tensed inside from the betrayal, anger and greed displayed by him and the English legal process, the pain became more and more violent and unbearable. Until that time I never could have imagined how severe menstrual pain could be. Only after I left England and recovered in the peace of my mountain home in Colorado was I able to relax my inner pelvis through dance and exercise, apply herbal and naturopathic treatments, and heal myself from this debilitating condition. I have now completely recovered and experience very little discomfort during my monthly flow.

*Diet:* Vitamins B6 and E, and Evening Primrose oil.

*Herbs:* Use the Women's Periodic, Bowel Rejuvenator and Female Reproductive formulae together with White Willow bark for pain; use Pulsatilla, Yarrow, Hops, Chasteberry, Black Cohosh, Motherwort and Oregon Grape root; it is essential to activate the liver and digestive processes whenever there is endometriosis as well as the entire systemic inner ecology; use progesterone herbs to balance the estrogen dependent endometriosis. Herbs can be taken in three phases to help balance the hormones and relieve the stress of endometriosis, using one formula during the period, one from the end of menses until the fourteenth day, or ovulation, and one formula from the fifteenth day to the start of the period, as described below.

1. Herbs to take during the monthly flow to balance hormones, relieve endometriosis, reduce pain and cramping and relax the nervous system: Black Haw, Chasteberry, False Unicorn root, Motherwort, Pulsatilla, Valerian, Vervain and Yarrow.

2. Estrogen formula to be taken after the monthly flow is over until ovulation: Alfalfa, Angelica, Black Cohosh, Borage, Oregon Grape root, Dong Quai, Hops, Licorice, Milk Thistle, Motherwort, Sage and Yellow Dock.

3. Progestrone Formula to be taken after ovulation until the monthly flow begins: Black Haw, Borage, Chasteberry, Dandelion, Lady's Mantle, Motherwort, Pulsatilla, Sarsaparilla, Vervain and Wild Yam.

*Homeopathy:* Take flower essences for emotional conditions and consult a homeopath.

*Therapies:* Emotional counseling, deep body work, pelvic relaxation and purification should be supported by a full individual treatment plan from *Herbs of Grace*.

My dear friend, Sandra, the artist who created the painting included in the Diamond Menopause section, that also graces the cover of *Herbs of Grace*, had such an amazing experience when she read the endometriosis section that I wish to include it here:

"Reading this page caused me to experience ghosts of pain/aching in my pelvic region and then rivers of tears came. Memories of endless therapies that didn't heal me, administered by cold, aloof doctors and cranky nurses, brought up anger and feelings of being deceived. Then, came the heartache and grieving for my lost womb and ovary. I felt as though I'd been invaded and robbed of my most prized possession, the symbol of my femininity. It was very painful to continue reading, but I understood the release of these emotions was beneficial for my healing. I closed my eyes and went inside to visit the cavity of my wound. I massaged my scar and told my body I was sorry I had allowed the mutilation to happen, but that I had simply not known any better at the time. I felt I wanted to fill up the dark empty space to repay my body for its loss. When I thought this – suddenly I saw in my mind's eye a beautiful glowing white lotus blossoming inside me where my womb used to be. I then visualized a lotus bud and curving stem to replace my fallopian tube and ovary. Then I visualized myself having a beautiful little silken cocoon in place of my appendix that was taken during my hysterectomy. The cocoon curled open and a gorgeous butterfly emerged and sat like a sentry guarding the gate between my small and large intestines. The lovely little butterfly began licking the wounded area where my appendix had been removed without my permission during my hysterectomy. I realized she was lubricating the area of my intestines that is normally lubricated with a healing fluid by the appendix. Once the vision ended, the tears stopped and I felt whole and safe for the first time since my operation in 1976. The tension and tight muscles I usually carry in my pelvis were gone – the aching pain was gone. The lower abdomen felt soft and full and free. The muscles felt relaxed and receptive instead of tense and protective. It was a marvelous healing experience. Thank you.

"P.S. I had endometriosis for over ten years and finally, desperately wanting to be free of pain, had a hysterectomy at age twenty-seven, fifteen years ago."

## EXHAUSTION & FATIGUE

Chronic fatigue, exhaustion, apathy, lack of energy and low metabolism can be part of the aging and menopausal picture. These debilitating symptoms can come in cycles or be part of a long–term chronic condition. First determine if there is hypothyroidism, toxicity, immune deficiency, constipation, insomnia, stress, overeating or overwork, and address these causes first. Treatment for fatigue can be approached from many different angles. Full constitutional support is essential, as is complete activation of all eliminative organs. Mental and emotional states together with difficult life conditions in work and marriage must also be faced and cleared because energy that is diverted to contain repressed emotions also contributes to exhaustion. Energy is activated and increased by spirituality, love, joy, creativity and a sense of purpose.

From time to time we may experience an energy slump or exhaustion. Using the methods described here, accept the exhaustion and move through the cycle, giving time and attention to loving self–care, herbs, diet, rest and treatment. Periods of exhaustion are also times of inner processing, release of deep emotions or adjustments in evolutionary processes. Tune in and go with the exhaustion. Life isn't always about jumping out of bed every morning and running around being active. Learn to enjoy the low energy times for the slowness, inner concentration and focus on being rather than doing. Listen for the message of the exhaustion and adjust life accordingly. Don't keep pushing as this will only cause deeper fatigue and illness.

Change the pace of life. Slow down. Appreciate leisure. Focus on the eternal rather than the ephemeral. The energy savings account of youth has been used up and now our energy comes from balance, ease, peace, good living habits, rest, relaxation and wholesome nourishing food.. Enjoyment of life and cooperation with the movement of the soul as it returns to its source also increases our energy when we regard our life journey as an adventure. Fear, attachment, frustration, desire and grief deplete our energy reserves.

*Diet:* Simple organic whole foods; fresh vegetable juices daily; eat seaweeds and the mono and purification, alkaline, vegetarian diets; avoid all preservatives, dyes and chemicals.

*Herbs:* Use the Exhaustion, Pancreas and Anemia herbal formulae; high iron herbs such as Yellow Dock energize the metabolism; thyroid herbs balance metabolic activity; blood purifiers and highly nutritive herbs such as Alfalfa and seaweeds also support recovery from exhaustion.

*Homeopathy:* Use Bach Flower essences *Olive* and *Hornbeam for fatigue*; *Gorse* can also be useful.

*Therapies:* Avoid beauty and home products which are not organic and natural; wear and sleep under natural fabrics, never use electric blankets; examine all aspects of home and work life to eliminate sources of energy drain from electricity, computers, overhead power cables, underground water, dampness, and lack of sunshine and fresh air; systemic cleansing increases energy.

## FIBROIDS, TUMORS & CYSTS

Abnormal growths are commonly associated with potassium deficiency, toxicity and lack of normal circulation of blood and lymph. These causes are influenced at deeper levels by mental attitudes, emotions, and lifestyle. The deep internal pain that often accompanies excess bleeding forces a woman's attention on her womb. While it may seem expedient to have the feminine organs removed, conscious self-healing of the entire life dynamic will bestow great gifts on women who are successful at releasing the need for such a condition.

Hormone dependent, nonmalignant fibroid tumors often disappear after the monthly flow ceases, except when women take estrogen replacement. The usual medical treatment is a hysterectomy, but herbs, purification, and other natural treatments can shrink fibroids.

Although benign, these fibroids cause disturbances such as pressure on other pelvic organs, constipation, flooding, back pain and menstrual difficulties. Small ones usually cause little disturbance, but large ones, which can be the size of a grapefruit, may cause major discomforts and may be difficult to shrink. Begin early. Don't let them grow. Ask what is growing in the womb that can't be released or brought into reality. Is the fibroid collecting negativity that can't be expressed? Ask for the truth of the fibroid's purpose. Make it conscious. Clear the need to have such a condition. They are often associated with relationship frustrations and infertility.

*Diet:* Make a daily meal of potassium broth: simmer potatoes, celery, carrots, onions and herbs; drink fresh vegetable juices; whole grains containing lignins are most abundant in flax seed, and less so in rye, buckwheat, millet, soya, oats, barley, corn, and rice; seaweeds, peas, soybeans, bananas, apple cider vinegar, and potassium supplements are excellent sources of potassium.

*Herbs:* Elderberry and flowers and Black Walnut are the highest sources of potassium; also useful are Black Currant buds or leaves, Chamomile, Corn silk, Chasteberry, Cramp bark, Garlic, Gromwell herb or seeds, Lady's Mantle, Yarrow flowers, Slippery Elm, Wild Carrot or Wild Pansy flowers; take the Female Reproductive formula three times daily; avoid Dong Quai which can increase fibroid size; Cotton root stops flooding due to fibroids: take one–half cup of the infusion or a dropper full of the tincture every five to ten minutes, until the strong bleeding stops.

*Homeopathy:* Use *Apis, Bryonia,* or *Lycopodium.*

*Therapies:* Apply Castor oil packs over the abdomen and where there are fibroids or cysts; Ginger kidney poultices help to activate elimination and strengthen the adrenals; acupuncture is useful to increase energy and strengthen the system; Slippery Elm and Comfrey poultices soften and nourish any area where there is hardening under the surface; they are recommended to be used directly over the abdominal area until the condition clears; a complete systemic purification and regeneration, and a three–month bowel cleansing program is necessary for best results.

## GUM & TEETH PROBLEMS

Loose teeth, pyorrhea, spongy gums, gum pockets and infections are the result of hormone imbalances, saliva changes, lack of proper tooth and gum care, aging and improper diet. After dealing with the constitutional, eliminative and nutritional aspects, try these specific remedies in conjunction with the total inner ecological treatment described in *Herbs of Grace*.

*Diet:* Eat fresh, organic, vegetarian fruits and vegetables, grains, nuts, seeds, and high calcium foods including almonds, sesame seeds, seaweeds and soybeans; eliminate all meat from the diet.

*Herbs:* Press a poultice made from White Oak bark mixed with Slippery Elm and water between the lips and gums of the upper and lower teeth every night until improvement is obtained; press the mixture into a moldable sports mouth guard for treatment on both sides of the teeth, upper and/or lower; other herbs for teeth and gums are Barberry, Bistort, Cranesbill, Myrrh, Oregon Grape and Prickly Ash; rub clove oil on teeth and gums whenever there is pain; take the Calcium formula regularly; drink Nettles and Horsetail tea daily; use herbal tinctures of Myrrh, Golden Seal and White Oak bark on the ends of toothpicks that are used to press into loose gums and gum pockets; soak a small amount of cotton batten in any of the recommended tinctures and press down inside a gum pocket while sleeping; also use the tinctures on toothbrushes, and in water used in dental cleansing equipment; gargle and swish diluted chlorophyll around the mouth to disinfect and nourish teeth and gums; apply a wheatgrass poultice over the gums.

*Homeopathy:* Use *Agave* for bleeding gums; *Alumina* for sore and bleeding gums; *Arsenicum* for unhealthy, easily bleeding gums; *Mercurius* for spongy, receding gums that bleed easily; *Phosphorus* for ulcerated, swollen bleeding gums.

*Therapies:* Make sure daily dental care is adequate; visit a dental hygienist twice or three times yearly as well as a dentist, and visit a periodontist at the first sign of gum trouble.

## HAIR BREAKING & HAIR LOSS

Hair problems are a concern during the aging process as graying hair changes texture, strength and color due to nutritional chemistry changes, calcium shortages, stress, circulation difficulties and digestive weaknesses that cause insufficient nutrition to the scalp and hair. Lack of exercise also limits cerebral circulation. The liver malfunctions, blood thickens, and circulation slows down contributing to hair weakness and loss. The extensive use of wheatgrass juice has been known to rejuvenate the body to such a degree that natural colored hair grows back.

*Diet:* Avoid heated oils, fats, fried foods, and high cholesterol foods like eggs, alcohol and junk foods; take in high minerals regularly by including seaweeds and herbs that build healthy hair.

*Herbs:* Use herbal hair washes; take the Cerebral Circulation and Calcium formulae internally; add Horsetail, an herb rich in silica, into daily herbal beverages.

*Homeopathy:* Use *Mercury, Nitricum Acidum* and *Silica,* and *Silica* tissue salts.

*Therapies:* Massage the head regularly, using natural oils and herbs which are rubbed into the scalp and left on all night; hair should be washed less often; massage the head reflexes on all the toes; take daily walks; exercise regularly; low impact aerobics increase circulation to the head.

### HEADACHES & MIGRAINES

Headaches during mid–life are most often liver related, due to the stress on this organ from hormonal changes and other digestive disorders affected by the hypothalamus. Severe headaches or migraines occur when there is a decrease of estrogen during the luteal and menstrual phases of the estrogen cycle. They also occur when estrogen–containing contraceptives have been discontinued, because estrogen increases vasomotor tone, thus inhibiting migraine tendencies. Migraines also result from dilation and distention of extracranial vessels, as well as from trigger foods such as alcohol, chocolate and drugs, combined with stress and cycle changes.

*Diet:* Avoid fats, fried foods, alcohol, cheese and chocolate; take vegetable juice fasts regularly and the liver cleanse drink for breakfast; try the mono diet to discover which foods may be aggravating the headaches; drink adequate water.

*Herbs:* Use the Liver/Gall Bladder formula, and liver herbs such as Gentian and Milk Thistle, the Circulatory formula to stimulate blood circulation, the Bowel Vitalizer or Rejuvenator formulae to cleanse and rejuvenate the gastrointestinal tract, and the Stomach/Acid Alkaline formula to improve digestion; take a drop of Peppermint aromatherapy oil in a cup of honey water to relieve headaches.

*Homeopathy:* Use *Cimicifuga, Cinchona, Ferrus, Ignacia, Lachesis, Sanguinaria* and *Sepia.*

*Therapies:* Apply the Castor oil pack over the liver; give deep massage to the reflexology foot points for the liver, head and neck; useful support can be received from polarity therapy, acupuncture, cranial sacral osteopathic adjustments, aromatherapy baths and oils, pressure points, rest and exercise; herbal or coffee enemas will stimulate bile flow and help to relieve the system immediately, especially if it is administered when the headache first comes on; rub Peppermint oil on the forehead, or drop it on a handkerchief or tissue and hold to the nose and head, especially when headaches are caused by digestive distress; sleep on Lavender or Neroli aromatherapy scented pillows; apply the full purification and rejuvenation program over three to six months to clear deep causes; when posture is a consideration take Alexander technique sessions to remove movement habits that affect the position of the head and neck. This work also helps to balance physical work stresses, spinal alignment and muscular tensions which may contribute to headaches.

## HEART PROBLEMS

More women die of heart disease than any other illness. Heart weakness is caused by the excessive intake of fats and oils, liver malfunction, increased toxicity levels and poor quality of blood. Mid–life is a time to evaluate our health, change patterns and take care of ourselves so that we can enjoy our old age. It is essential to support liver function, keep the blood clean and fluid, keep the bowels moving, move the lymph through exercise, keep blood pressure normal, and use dietary therapy, herbs and exercise to keep fit so that we can avoid heart disease. Consider the Circulatory Hardening iris constitutional type in *Herbs of Grace*, which informs us of heart and circulatory weakness through lacunae, radii soleris, abnormal colors and reflexive fibers in the iris heart and circulatory areas.

Caution: Estrogen replacement therapy (ERT) raises blood pressure, increases blood clotting and the levels of triglycerides; hormone replacement therapy (HRT) increases risks of strokes and heart attacks.

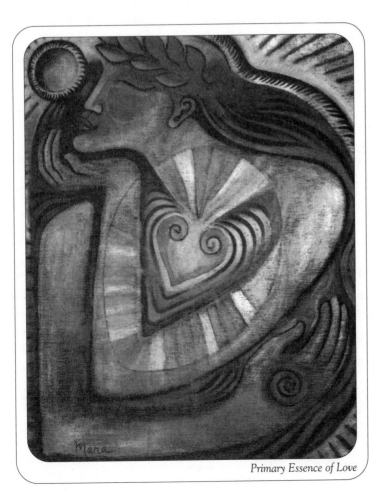

*Primary Essence of Love*

*Diet:* Avoid fats, cooked oils, eggs, margarine, ice cream and fried foods; take essential fatty acids in vitamin E, flax, Black Currant, Borage or wheat germ oils; use lecithin and buckwheat to thin cholesterol in the blood; take niacin (500mg with food three times a day), and vitamins C and E; Garlic, raw or lightly cooked, lowers blood pressure, reduces cholesterol and phospholipids, helps prevent platelet clumping and clotting and stabilizes blood sugar.

*Herbs:* Use the Heart and Circulation formulae; Hawthorn berries (chew one a day) are an excellent heart tonic; Motherwort lowers blood pressure, eases palpitations and irregularities and strengthens the heart; Lemon Balm also strengthens the heart; use Alfalfa, Bedstraw, Buckwheat, Birch, Red Clover, White Willow and Wintergreen to thin the blood; high amounts of Cayenne increase circulation and relieve heart pain both therapeutically and during emergencies.

*Therapies: Use* flower essences, reflexology, acupuncture, chiropractic or osteopathy treatments to relieve spinal stress and misalignment in the thoracic area; do not smoke or allow excess weight and water to collect; take exercise every day; develop the heart center by practicing giving and receiving; open your heart and clear and release any wounds of the heart; ask for hugs and give hugs; have regular massages, especially if you are not in a relationship; touch and be touched; reiki and polarity therapy also help to balance the heart center.

## HOT FLASHES & NIGHT SWEATS

Hot flashes occur due to changing estrogen levels. The more toxic or the more unbalanced we are through repressed or excessive emotions, stress and mental pressure, the more acute and uncomfortable the flashes are, sometimes continuing during sleep hours as night sweats.

On another level they are messages from the unconscious, bringing up blocked sexual and emotional energy for release and deepening our insight as we face our repressed, denied and unborn selves. It is my experience that hot flashes lessen and eventually stop as the body, mind and spirit return to balance. They often signal the initiation aspect of menopause. Hot flashes can also be enjoyed and celebrated as flames of the greater flame of transformation.

Flashes can be triggered and accentuated by hot, acidic foods and drinks, caffeine, alcohol, sugar, meat fats, hot temperatures, hot baths, saunas, tobacco, excessive physical exercise and sexual stimulation and hot fiery feelings such as jealousy, anger and possessiveness.

*Diet:* Add soy beans, yams, whole grains and seaweeds to the daily diet; take vitamin E, royal jelly and Evening Primrose oil.

*Herbs:* Black Cohosh, which is high in phytosterols, effectively relieves hot flashes, as does Dong Quai, Blessed Thistle, False Unicorn, Ginseng and Sarsaparilla; drink Fenugreek tea on waking and before sleep; liver herbs such as Milk Thistle, Dandelion and Yellow Dock also help to relieve flashes; Chickweed stabilizes the glandular temperature control system; Elderflower cools body temperature and reduces hot flashes – it is the youth element, the highest source of potassium, and it benefits skin and hair and energy; Violet cools the flashes and reduces cancer risk; other useful herbs include any of the mallows and mints, and Hibiscus; use Sage, Motherwort and Oatstraw as well as adrenal herbs or formulae to reduce and eliminate night sweats; make or buy natural progesterone creams made from Wild Yam, and apply daily for prevention as well as during hot flashes.

*Homeopathy:* Use *Nux Vomica* for night sweats and leg cramps; *Sulfur* for night sweats accompanied by thirst and intolerance of heat; *Crotalus* relieves severe flashing with headaches, flooding, restlessness, weakness; *Caladium* when there is itching.

*Therapies: Take* Scullcap and Chickweed baths before bed to calm the system, decrease night sweats and reduce the discomfort of itching that often accompanies hot flashes.

## INSOMNIA

Insomnia is usually the end result of a combination of different aging and menopausal symptoms: pain, aches, liver disorders, digestive disorders, emotions, anxiety, hot flashes, night sweats, chills and anxiety. Medical drugs relieve the condition but do not address the cause.

*Diet:* Eat as early as possible in the evening and exercise before sleep.

*Herbs:* Take the Sweet Sleep formula and drink Valerian infusion before bed; drink Horsetail tea during the day; take high Calcium supplements or herbs; Chamomile or Catnip enemas are calming and relaxing and Lobelia baths provide deep relaxation.

*Homeopathy: Coffea, Cypripedium, Ignatia, Passiflora, Aquilegia; White Chestnut* and *Mimulus* are useful Bach flower remedies.

*Therapies:* Aromatherapy baths, herbal baths, massage, reflexology, music, relaxation tapes, meditation, and visualization will help relieve insomnia; meditation is the ultimate remedy.

## OSTEOPOROSIS

Osteoporosis has become one of the greatest fears women have about the menopause transition because of modern medical propaganda. This condition is caused by lack of, and/or poor calcium assimilation, which requires the synergistic minerals phosphorus and silica. It is also affected by thyroid and parathyroid functions that govern calcium metabolism. These glands in the throat center are related to the ether element and excessive grief and longing, imbalances of which also influence the development of this condition, as does fear that is associated with the earth element. The stress of modern life and the tensions it creates within us are also a major contributors to this condition. This condition is rare in third world countries.

The digestive system must be working efficiently enough to digest and assimilate natural calcium when it is available. Acid blood invites osteoporosis. The parathyroids will remove calcium from the bones to balance the blood pH. Blood acidity is caused by acid foods, excess meat protein, stress, strong emotions, anxiety and the buildup of toxins in the body. Truly, osteoporosis is a systemic condition which requires women to track down the individual causes in our lives and treat the condition in a holistic way.

Bone loss and calcium depletion begin before mid–life due to stress, poor diet, over–exercising and anorexia. This loss is not caused just by the menopausal hormonal changes because bone is a dynamic, constantly renewing body tissue that is affected by all aspects of our being. Progesterone also helps to build new bones. It is important for menopausal women to allow a reasonable amount of increase in natural body fat that will support estrogen production, because excessive thinness reduces natural hormones and helps begin bone dissolution early in life.

A bone growth pause follows menopause for about five years. During this time bones reject calcium and bone loss increases. It is important to prepare for this time by increasing the amounts of natural vegetarian sources of calcium during premenopausal and menopausal years, and decreasing the amounts of high protein meat and junk foods.

Early warning signs of calcium deficiency are night cramps in feet and legs, gum and tooth problems, periodontal gum disease, loose teeth, insomnia, backache and loss of height.

Calcium deficiency is a major contributor to bone loss. When more bone cells die than are created, the aging process of osteoporosis has begun and bone mass loss begins. Eating calcium and other mineral rich natural foods and supplements, and taking regular exercise, helps prevent this process. One of the main arguments for taking (ERT) estrogen replacement therapy is to slow down bone loss, but this not only increases risk of cancer, it is also expensive. Prepare for menopause by building your bones before age forty.

The parathyroid endocrine glands monitor calcium levels in the blood and secrete hormones to balance and keep optimum levels. Excess calcium is stored in bones, the soft tissue or joints. When there is a shortage, the parathyroid glands stimulate calcium release from the bones, inducing loss of bone mass.

Be gentle, but consistent, with exercise. Keep the blood moving through the bones. Keep life energy circulating without force, stress or strain.

*Diet:* Oatmeal, seaweeds, tahini, tofu, yogurt, blackstrap molasses, leafy greens should be included in the diet, as well as a daily drink of apple cider vinegar and honey to improve digestion and any hydrochloric acid deficiency; soak one cup of pre–soaked and rinsed organic wheat for forty-eight hours in three cups of water, and drink it every day to provide the fermentation necessary to help restore intestinal flora; soak almonds overnight, peel, and eat as a calcium rich source of nutrient; beta carotene (50,000 units) increases progesterone and aids bones; avoid excess salt and protein, which increases the loss of calcium through urine; avoid high oxalic acid greens such as rhubarb, spinach, beet greens, chard and sorrel; also avoid soda, white flour, meat, junk food, coffee, alcohol and white flour products, and processed foods which increase calcium loss and diminish calcium production; take calcium–rich foods in natural synergy and eventually the bones will accept calcium again; natural magnesium, manganese, boron, vitamin D, zinc, copper, folic acid, and silica are all necessary ingredients for healthy bones; read the *Herbs of Grace* list for natural food and herbal sources for all the vitamins and minerals necessary for good health; vitamin K is required for the production of osteocalcin, the key calcium–binding matrix protein involved in bone mineralization.

*Herbs:* Use the Calcium formula regularly as well as individual herbs that are high in calcium, such as Horsetail, Nettles, and Dandelion leaves, and Fenugreek for Vitamin D; make sure natural progesterone is available by using Wild Yam in powder or as an ointment.

*Homeopathy:* Use *Silica* tissue salts, *Symphytum*; Bach Flower remedies, *Mimulus*, *Aspen* and *Rock Water* are useful for the earth element of the bones, and its accompanying emotion of fear.

*Therapies:* Take regular air and sunbaths; wear comfortable flat shoes; walk carefully; do balancing yoga postures; the discriminate gentle use of leg and arm weights is helpful, as are other weight–bearing exercises; get to know your bones, nails, teeth and hair by interior visualization; play or listen to cello or drum music and let it vibrate the bones; bones are support and structure; communicate with the earth element and release the emotion of fear; develop the inner life with prayer and meditation; seek out the wise ones, the elders, the spiritual teachers and the survivors to teach, guide and inspire you; release the negative pole of the earth element through polarity therapy and clear fixation stress by restoring flexibility and mutability.

## PMS – PREMENSTRUAL SYDROME

PMS symptoms vary from woman to woman and can include: sore breasts, alternating constipation or diarrhea, digestive gas, water retention, bloating and emotional sensitivity or excesses. Premenstrual symptoms can also occur after miscarriage, childbirth, abortion, surgery or an unpleasant or violent sexual encounter. Injuries, infections and spinal displacement caused by the above also need to be treated to help improve the condition. Low–grade pelvic infections should not be suppressed with antibiotics. The cause should be eliminated by bowel cleansing and lymphatic activation. Both toxins and inflammatory conditions may exist in the pelvis. A thorough systemic purification and regeneration treatment is essential to clear the cause as well as the condition.

*Diet:* Observe which foods are craved before the onset of the monthly flow and balance the cravings with herbs and supplements; eat foods high in natural progesterone during the two weeks before the flow: soybeans, Wild Yam, and Evening Primrose oil; avoid alcohol, chocolate, caffeine, cigarettes, fried foods and white sugar.

*Herbs:* To reduce PMS use progesterone herbs, Alfalfa, Chasteberry, Lady's Mantle, Pulsatilla; Sarsaparilla, Wild Yam and Yarrow; nourish the nervous system with Nerve Rejuvenator and Vitalizer formulae, and adrenals with Borage and the Adrenal formula; detoxify the liver with

Dandelion, Barberry and Milk Thistle; stimulate bowel cleansing with Licorice or either of the bowel formulae; apply natural progesterone creams made from Wild Yam root on a daily basis, as well as more often during PMS; leave Oregon Grape root out of any progesterone formula.

*Homeopathy:* Use *Sanguinaria* for enlarged, painful breasts; *Ignacia* for hysteria; *Cimicifuga* for mental depression or irritability; *Pulsatilla* for a weepy changeable nature together with distended abdomen and diarrhea during menses; *Bryonia* for breast tenderness.

*Therapies:* Clear unfinished emotional problems through communication before the onset of the menses; take time to rest and be alone; let tears flow. Have a massage just before the flow is due; ask for hugs; talk to someone who will listen; release anger or frustration through exercise, therapy and flower remedies; keep the bowels clear and active.

## SKIN DISCOLORATION

Liver related skin discoloration and spots often occur during aging. This is due to increased stress, excessive emotions, toxicity, poor diet, pollution, drugs, chemicals, dyes, and preservatives which cause unhealthy changes in body chemistry. Hundreds of natural medicine clients over the years experienced their spots fading when their liver was rejuvenated with diet and herbal programs, and their bodies relieved by purification treatment. The marks can be removed by a dermatologist with a simple spray, but that does not deal with the cause. The important factor here is that this is the sign that it is time to detoxify and rejuvenate the liver, and take care with exposure to the sun. Full systemic treatment is recommended.

## VAGINAL CHANGES

Thinning of vaginal walls and drying due to lower amounts of vaginal lubrication often accompany menopause because of decreasing levels of estrogen. Estrogen Replacement Therapy is the usual medical treatment. However it is important to consider the potential side effects and consider alternative natural treatment first. Keep your life lubricated, flexible and young in spirit. Strengthen the adrenals and the nervous system, and become determined to complete a three–to six–month purification and regeneration treatment.

*Diet:* Eat potassium foods; eat pomegranates, soybeans and alfalfa sprouts for natural estrogen; eliminate alcohol, tobacco, carbonated drinks and sugar; take vitamin E and Evening Primrose oil.

*Herbs:* Whenever decreased vaginal lubrication and thinning of the vaginal membranes occurs, take Elderflower tincture for natural potassium; take internally or make douches and ointments from high estrogen herbs such as Dong Quai, Horsetail, Black Cohosh, Hops, Licorice and Sage; add Calendula, Comfrey and St. Joan's Wort for healing properties; natural progesterone of Wild Yam when it is made into an ointment also relieves vaginal dryness; a soothing paste made by mixing Aloe Vera with Slippery Elm will also provide natural lubrication.

*Homeopathy:* Aconite, Apis, Belladonna, Lycopodium or Nat. Mur. are useful for vaginal dryness.

*Therapies:* Visualize a healthy, moist vagina; concentrate on quality instead of quantity in your sexual life; avoid using chemical contraceptives, creams and douches, and use natural oils for lubrication such as Coconut oil, wheat germ or vitamin E oil, and any pure food oils such as almond, apricot, avocado and jojoba oils; honey is also a natural spermicide.

## WATER RETENTION

When women's bodies become heavier during the change of life, problems may arise due to water retention, which is the result of imbalances in hormonal cycles, the kidney, adrenal and lymphatic systems, constitutional weakness, improper dietary habits, and emotional distress. Different climates also affect our bodies, influencing both a shortage or excess of fluids. Exercise plays an important part in moving lymphatic fluids that cause congestion and water retention in the ankles, thighs and hips. Female bodies reveal repressed and unprocessed emotions when they retain water in the thighs and hips. The body tends to slim down when the emotional content is released and completed. A deeper understanding and relationship with the water element and its different moods and dimensions as expressed in sexuality, desire, attraction and repulsion, deep feelings, and instincts, will help to make more conscious of the emotional aspect of water retention. Excess water will put out the elemental fire energy of change and transformation. An increase of fire energy transforms excess water. We recommend an iris analysis to determine the individual constitutional type and the condition of immune system.

*Diet:* Become conscious of daily fluid intake, and drink less or more as needed; go on a ten–day diet of high amounts of brown rice chewed slowly with baked vegetables; drink only two cups of water a day, swish the water in the mouth to relieve thirst, then swallow or spit out; eliminate salt entirely, or use very little; natural diuretic foods are asparagus, celery, corn, cucumber, grapes, parsley, and watermelon; cranberry juice is a specific aid for the urinary system; avoid mucus forming and acidic foods, and all foods and drinks that contain preservatives, chemicals, dyes and sugar; dietary changes are essential; the purification, mono, alkaline, vegetarian and juice diets are most effective for both quick and long lasting results.

*Herbs:* The Kidney/Bladder, Lymphatic and Anti-Weight and Water formulae, together with the Waterbalance tea, are useful for this condition; Dandelion removes excess fluid from the cells and nourishes and tones the adrenals, kidneys and liver; Nettle nourishes the kidneys and adrenals; Bladderwrack helps eliminate excess weight and water; Juniper aromatherapy oil baths and massage stimulate natural diuretic action; if the water and weight are mostly on the lower half of the body, take therapeutic herbal or aromatherapy hip baths regularly; when depression and overeating are part of the condition, use Clary Sage or Ylang Ylang aromatherapy baths; to help thin hips and thighs, and reduce cellulite, make a massage oil using equal parts of Cypress and Juniper oils in a vegetable oil base, and apply twice daily with a vigorous stimulating motion.

*Homeopathy:* Use *Apis* for swelling, dropsy, edema; use *Arsenica* for itching, burning swelling, especially on the feet and ankles; *Crab Apple* and *Agrimony* are useful Bach flower remedies.

*Therapies:* Apply the Ginger poultice to both kidneys once a week, or more often if needed, to increase their strength and circulation; massage and exercise are essential; receive emotional release therapies such as polarity and hakomi.

## WEIGHT GAIN & LOSS

Weight gain is a natural part of aging. Because fat cells produce estrogens, heavier women often have an easier, more gradual, menopause change, with less discomfort from hot flashes and other symptoms. Enjoy, admire and respect the full-bodied woman with the ripe rich beauty of maturity. Love your full, ripe self. Dismiss the thin myth as it does not serve you, but also take care to avoid obesity and its many problems. Strive for balance. Practice releasing affirmations.

*Diet:* To lose weight, drink two cups of fresh soy milk daily; take flax seed oil and wheat germ oil; eat olives, wild greens, oatmeal, wheatgrass and barley greens; it is also important to avoid starches, sugars and fats; do not drink either too much or too little liquid; strive for moderation.

*Herbs:* Natural safe weight loss can be achieved by using Bladderwrack, in six to twelve capsules dosage per day, or drink two cups of Bladderwrack tea a day for up to three months; Chickweed is also effective as is the regular use of alfalfa, spirulina, seaweeds together with Nettles and Hops herbs, and the Anti-Weight and Water herbal formula.

*Homeopathy:* Use *Fucus* for thyroid related obesity; *Phytolacca* to decrease weight.

*Therapies:* Regular brisk walking, cycling and swimming, tai chi, and yoga move fluids through the body, and trim and tone the muscles; aerobics are valuable as long as they are not overdone; it is essential to have enough body fat to help produce estrogen during and after menopause, without being overweight.

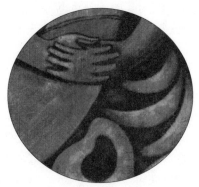

# Emotional Clearing

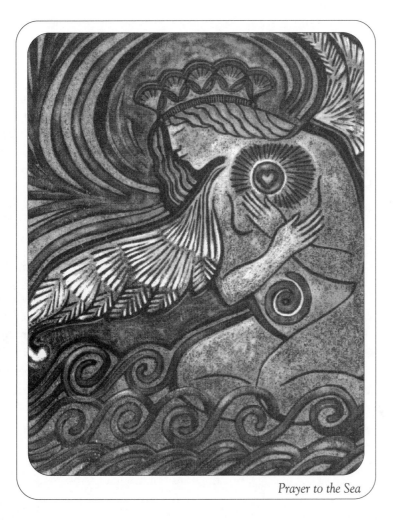

*Prayer to the Sea*

Weeding the garden of our lives is an essential task of maturity. As our consciousness expands, discrimination becomes refined and responsibility takes on deeper meaning. Clearing the weeds, thorns and thistles from our hearts and feelings frees us to experience the bliss of higher mind and spirituality. Although we long for the grace of unconditional love we find our desires, our fears and our power issues make this impossible. Our cherished emotional wounds cling like a tattered cloth we cannot bear to part with. We are imprisoned in a secret garden that has turned into a briar patch. Our own thorns and thistles choke our capacity to give and receive love, and although we hold the promise of roses, lotuses and lilies they cannot flourish. We must dig out the roots of excessive and unbalanced elemental emotions that pull us into negativity. We must tame, nourish and channel the gifts of the elements towards our highest purpose.

There is a growing body of humanistic psychology, New Age teachings, metaphysical mysteries and spirituality that offers inspiration, leadership and instruction on the many and various ways of freeing ourselves from our emotional bondage. As women we are very close to the sacred realities of life, birth and nurturing. Spirituality waits to bloom in the garden of our lives, once we have cleared the thorns and thistles from its path. Explore, seek and persevere until the path opens. Daily practice and continuous clearing will help reap the harvest our hearts long for.

Carl Jung left a body of work to show us how to become whole and fulfilled by integrating what he defined as 'the unconscious shadow of denial and repression.' He named this process of integration and maturation 'Individuation.' During my menopause I experienced within my own being the truths of what he organized into his psychological system. Although each woman's experience is unique, it is helpful to understand the process. I invite you to explore his work and that of many of his students and colleagues who have expanded into deeper and wider creativity from the seeds that he has sown.

If the change of life is upon us, let us cooperate with change by trying new ways of living and being. Let us take the opportunity and the freedom to become what we have not been before. Instead of growing toward maturity, we are now preparing for a greater life, the life of the spirit. This requires that we begin to focus on the internal life as we willingly release the outer. The more slowly we do this, and the more time and energy we devote to the process, the easier it will be to let go of this world gracefully, and with a sense of completion, when our time comes. Aging and death become an enriching experience as we attune to the part of our being that is growing and developing at the same time that our physical body is fading from this world. We no longer need a man, another person or a mirror to show us how beautiful we are. We are beautiful within. Let us connect with our refined spiritual essence within and let that beauty radiate, shine and expand as we let go of our attachment to what we believe we should look like and who we think we are, and let ourselves become what we truly are, our spiritual selves, our true, complete, fulfilled, realized higher selves. This is a true release from co–dependency as we draw meaning and become nourished from within ourselves.

Clearing and freeing our emotional lives is a necessary part of the menopausal transition into the second half of our lives. During the transition we must strive to clear, release and let go of all suppressed, unfinished and denied emotions, to free ourselves for truthful expression and cosmic creativity. It is essential that women keep their balance during the release because excessive emotional indulgence eventually leads to physical problems, as well as disturbing those around us. Body–centered therapy systems such as hakomi, polarity and rosenwork, psychotherapy, and dance and art therapy help clear emotional blockages and provide tools to process emotional distress. Menopause gives women the opportunity, and hopefully the time and space, to release, clear and make conscious the repressions, denials, or unfinished experiences that inhibit our expression of creativity and truth.

Once the layer of repressed and denied emotions have been released, the integration of the shadow deepens and expands our being, so that we can take the powerful negative emotions usually associated with aging and death and turn them around to focus on the eternal and the spiritual. Fear of the unknown can become very powerful. It can cause us to cling with excessive attachment to people, places, things as well as to our role of who we think we are. This causes us to contract as we hold on. We can feel tremendous anger at the aging process, and speed and greed can overtake us as we try to get and take all we can from life. Grief for what we are leaving behind can also be overwhelming if we only acknowledge this outward reality. Emptiness and boredom can inhibit us if we refuse to experience the aging process, and do not participate in the adventure of transformation.

Hysteria or emotional excesses such as weeping, sobbing, screaming, despair and obsession, all come from different combinations of the basic emotions of fear, attachment and desire, anger, speed and greed, and grief and longing. Because the feminine essence expresses itself more naturally in feelings and relationships, imbalances caused by external difficulties are usually expressed or repressed through emotional excesses or shortages.

The more the world and men resist women's feelings and truth, the more the women go out of balance, until strong and passionate emotions create chaos and illness in their lives. Hysterectomy comes from the root word hysteria. Surgeons believed that women's excessive emotions would be stopped if they removed the female organs. This is not the answer. The greatest healing women experience is achieved by getting deeply in touch with their feelings and developing the language and the ability to express their truth in a way that can be accepted and respected in this world. Instead of self destructing, our energy within can then be used for creativity, service and the highest purpose of our lives.

Dryness or emotional shortage is a condition of lack of feeling, together with an inability to express oneself or ask for help. Some escape into mental or business activities to avoid feeling. Others harden their hearts, or sink into depression, apathy or fear. Repression and denial causes natural human responses to freeze into nonfeeling. Because so much energy is used to contain unexpressed emotion, exhaustion and weakness result. Women close down to avoid pain, but the pain is still there in another form. We must open our internal lives without fear, shame or guilt, feel the pain and allow sensitive feelings to flower in this interior desert.

Bach flower remedies taken hourly for five days release blocked emotions, reduce excessive or indulgent emotions and awaken repressed emotions. The causes for emotional distress must be brought into the light of day. We may need to seek professional counselling. It is also important for friends and family to offer support, compassion, understanding and caring to help women pass through these storms so that they may emerge as wise women, balanced and free from emotional distress. For emotional shortages use *Star of Bethlehem*, *Wild Rose*, *Agrimony* and *Aspen* flower remedies to warm and melt the feeling water element from this frozen waste. Tears must flow. Emotions must be released. For excesses use *Vervain* for overreacting, *Rescue Remedy* whenever there are strong upsets, *Mimulus* and *Aspen* for fear, *Red Chestnut* and *Vine* for excessive attachment, *Holly*, *Impatiens* and *Willow* for anger and greed and *Star of Bethlehem* for grief.

Herbal treatments can relieve hysteria. Drink Catnip herbal tea and completely clear the bowels with Catnip enemas; retain the enema for five to ten minutes; repeat as necessary.

Homeopathy also offers support. *Ignacia* is a useful remedy for hysterical, excitable, sensitive natures that change and contradict, and that sob and sigh with grief and worry. More detailed treatment information is offered later in this section.

## THERAPEUTIC POSSIBILITIES
## FOR EMOTIONAL IMBALANCES & EXCESSES

*'Women need to be touched, held and listened to.'*

Love

Hugs

Body work

Creativity

Counseling

Singing

Dance

Color

Beauty

Travel

Nature

Solitude

Service

Meditation

Psychotherapy

Spiritual teachers

Women's Groups

Elemental Energetics

Cranial sacral balancing

Prayerful sweat lodges

Flower remedies and essences

# ELEMENTAL ENERGETICS

*'If you don't dance the elements, they dance you.'*

*Surrender*
as though you are the rose opening before the divine
to receive the gentle dew of bliss

*Focus*
as though you are a laser lighthouse manifesting authentic reality
and concentrating power to open the inner eye

*Empty*
as though you are infinite longing spreading like nectar
through your being

*Expand*
as though you are the atmosphere
achieving equilibrium, balance and contentment

*Seek*
as though you are the hungry flame
devouring fuel and achieving transformation

*Dive down*
as though you are the vast ocean
and free the movements of your sexuality and your soul

*Dig deep*
as though you are the abundant earth
and loosen your roots so that they may receive nourishment

# THE ELEMENTS OF LIFE

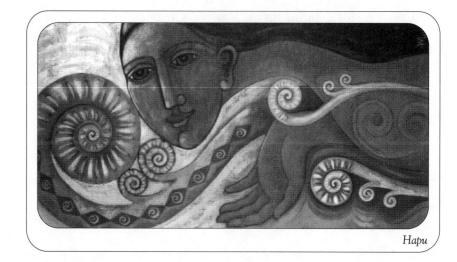

*Hapu*

The elements of life have been a part of every system of natural medicine and culture since the beginning of time. They are a fact of life that dances all around us in nature and more subtly within our physical, emotional, sexual, mental and spiritual bodies. They are the elemental forces with which we and this world are formed. When we are released from our physical bodies, the elements return to their source, earth to earth, water to water, fire to fire, air to air, ether to ether, while our souls fly free to seek union with the divine Soul, our original source.

All systems of medicine, from ancient Egyptian, Greek, Islamic, Roman, Ayurvedic and Chinese as well as indigenous cultures and shamanic healing, are all based on some organization of the elements of life. We will look at emotional imbalances and their causes in blocked elemental energies within our various body systems, organs, tissues, fluids and glands.

The seven chakras, or spinning wheels of energy, of the Yogic and Hindu religious traditions are also related to the elements of life – from the sacral root chakra which is earth, through reproductive water, digestive fire, heart and respiratory air, to the throat chakra which is the home of ether, the source of all the elements. These chakras correspond to physical nerve plexuses in the body as well as to subtle energy patterns. The elements that are related to the main emotions or passions are: earth fear, water desire and attachment, fire anger, air greed and ether grief. When the psyche is wanting to clear, let go and move upward to evolve, attain fulfillment and prepare for release and death, many old emotions and imbalances surface because they need to be completed and released. It is a time for intense growth which can be supported in creative ways. The passions are transformed into positive states of consciousness which support our personal, spiritual and evolutionary processes.

To learn more about the chakras, elements and emotions, you are invited to attend my workshops called Elemental Energetics – Movements of the Soul which explore these powerful, though seemingly invisible, realities and make them a valuable part of our conscious lives.

## EARTH ELEMENTAL FEAR OR SECURITY

FEAR – ANXIETY – INSECURITY – HOLDING ON
INABILITY TO MAKE CHANGES OR TAKE RISKS – RESISTANCE – DENIAL

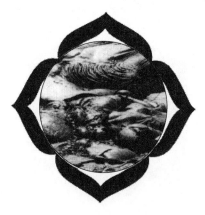

The earth element resides in the sacral plexus, and in the bones, teeth, hair, nails and the adrenals, which give the dynamic energy for flight or fight survival. The emotion associated with the earth element is fear. While it is healthy and good to have a certain amount of fear, awe, respect and uncertainty in order to keep our instincts and our skills alive, excess fear inhibits joy, creativity, change, love, truth and our unfoldment as a human and spiritual being. Fear also creates disease through the stiffening, hardening, crystallizing process of the earth element.

Fear takes many shapes and forms in our imagination, except when we are faced with an actual situation where we have three alternatives, fight, flight, or becoming a victim. When we get older our fear intensifies as we resist the idea of aging and death. Around this primal fear constellates many fears: of the unknown; of becoming wrinkled and ugly; of being useless and neglected; of pain and disease; of being helpless and poor; and of having no one to take care of us. When people are fearful they cling to what is known, whether it is good for them or not, and they use tremendous energy to build security through materialism. Through clinging and holding on to the past and not letting go and taking risks, they get stuck, harden, resist and miss opportunities that would bring about change, transformation and fulfillment.

Bone diseases, constipation, gall stones, kidney stones, hardening of the arteries and rigidity are associated with imbalances of the earth element.

A positive earth element provides security, stability, abundance and a structural foundation. We achieve balance that enables us to be both grounded and spiritual. We are able to enjoy the material world, but we are not excessively attached to it because we fear loss, change or death.

Useful Bach flower remedies for fear are: *Mimulus* for worry fears, *Aspen* for unknown fears, *Larch* for fearing the worst will happen, *Sweet Chestnut* for fearing loss of control and *White Chestnut* for the obsession with and the repetition of fears and anxieties in the mind.

# WATER ELEMENTAL DESIRE OR NURTURING

## ATTACHMENT – SEXUALITY – LUST – LACK OF FEELING – EXCESSIVE DESIRE
## ATTRACTION & REPULSION – SOCIAL DUTIES & ROLES

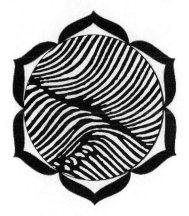

The water element resides in the reproductive plexus, the ovaries, womb and urinary organs, as well as in all the body fluids (blood, lymph, tears, mucus, urine, discharges, saliva and amniotic fluids). The emotion associated with the water element is desire, which creates movements toward or away from something due to attraction or repulsion. Social structures help us possess what we desire and control sexuality, procreation and lineage. This element is most often associated with the feminine essence.

Attachment is a different form of clinging to the past, to the way things are and were, to our children, to ideas that are no longer appropriate, to mates who have died, divorced or left, to images of ourself that have faded, to things or to memories. The present moment is wasted in imagination. The past is held in our mind, so the present and the future are diluted and impotent. The mental state is related to our being over–identified with our children, mate, friends and family, and being unable to let go of position, roles, finances and social structures. It is also related to sexual changes – desire, lust, frigidity and all the unfinished sexual experiences and longings we find are still strong in our mind and emotions. Lust can become so powerful in old age that it keeps us from peace, contentment, spirituality and personal fulfillment. Lust keeps us constantly hungry and dissatisfied because the more we get, the more we want. The abuse of young children is an example of how this energy can become perverse.

Reproductive and urinary diseases are associated with the water element as well as physical and emotional problems with sexuality, fertility and desire.

A balanced water element gives us the ability to access deep feeling, intuition and instinct. Freed from chaotic attraction and repulsion desires we perform our duties with respect and nurture and are nurtured by those we love and care for.

Useful Bach flower remedies are: *Vine* for control, *Red Chestnut* for excessive attachment to loved ones, and *Star of Bethlehem* for releasing attachment by attaining peace within.

# FIRE ELEMENTAL WILL OR TRANSFORMATION

ANGER – FRUSTRATION – JEALOUSY – PASSION – MANIPULATION
PERSONAL WILL – POWER STRUGGLES – LOSS OF POWER

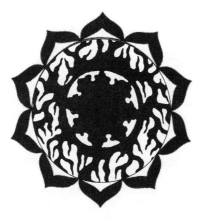

The fire element resides in the digestive plexus and locally in digestive organs and glands, in metabolic energy and warmth, and in the eyes. The emotions associated with the fire element are anger, will, jealousy and passion, which rise up like lava from a volcano to help us obtain what we want, regardless of the cost. Fire also causes change due to power struggles when people seek to dominate and use others and the environment to get what they want. This element is most often associated with the masculine essence.

As women our feminine nature is traditionally passive. We are conditioned from an early age to not get angry, to please, keep quiet, endure and be receptive. Without the deep interior levels of truth and intuition to guide us when we are impotent outwardly we become vassals and victims. Lost in the illusion that power is something from the outside, something that is given to us by a father or a husband, by position or youth, we lose the potential power of our elder status, and our nobility and wisdom. The present moment is wasted in useless frustration. Instead of using life experience and inner power to serve and contribute to the world, fulfill ourselves and develop our inner lives, we victimize ourselves by not taking our own power.

These negative fire emotions hold us back, but when we change to the positive fire flame of transformation, we become fed up, ready to leap, take the risk and change; we leave behind the downward weight of earth, water and fire negativity and move up to the heart where we are able to give and receive love without excessive emotion, desire or fear.

Digestive problems, especially those of liver, gall bladder, duodenum, pancreas and spleen, are associated with the fire elemental emotions, as well as body temperature mechanisms.

A balanced fire element gives us energy for change and transformation, for achieving goals in a respectful way, and for rising to the heart center of equilibrium and unconditional love.

Useful Bach flower remedies are: *Holly* for anger, *Willow* for resentment and blame, *Impatiens* for impatience, *Vine* for domination and control, *Centaury* for being unable to free ourselves from domination, and *Pine* for guilt.

# AIR ELEMENTAL SPEED & GREED OR EQUILIBRIUM

## LACK OF LOVE
### RESISTANCE TO GIVING & RECEIVING – BELIEVING THERE IS NEVER ENOUGH

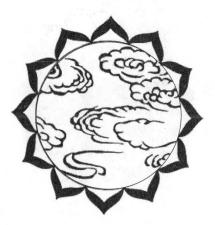

The air element resides in the heart center and the respiratory functions and organs (the lungs are also related to the ether element and the throat center). The emotion associated with the air element is love, which when out of balance, moves into speed and greed because we believe there isn't enough time, energy, wealth, love and resources to go around.

Air imbalances are created by focusing on what we do not have, by limiting love and by being unable to serve and give equally to all around us. By staying in a state of starvation where we believe that there is not enough of whatever we need or want, we waste the abundance of the present moment and relinquish the peaceful contentment of equilibrium and unconditional love. This unbalanced mental state is very common in this age of materialism.

Let go and open to abundance. We must learn to let love flow, to give and receive in truth, trust and love, so that we can experience the joy of balance and equilibrium in our lives. Because all the elements are contained in the blood – earth nutrients and minerals, water fluid, fire warmth, air oxygen and ether prana, the heart is affected by all the elements and in turn affects all the elements. The heart is in the center between the three lower chakras and their associated elements of earth, water and fire, and the three higher chakras of ether and the brow and crown chakras.

Heart, thymus, shoulder, arm and hand problems are associated with the air element, as well as breathing difficulties.

Positive air element energy spreads out in balance to achieve equilibrium in all aspects of being. This equality of attention enables us to give and receive love freely, to live in the present moment and to live in harmony with nature and other living beings.

Useful Bach flower remedies are: *Vervain* for overenthusiasm and excessive activity, *Elm* for being overwhelmed, and *Impatiens* for the impatience that accelerates speed and greed.

# ETHER ELEMENTAL GRIEF OR SPIRITUAL LONGING

## GRIEF – EMPTINESS – SORROW – LONGING – MELANCHOLY – DEPRESSION

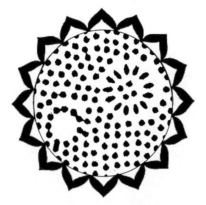

The ether element resides in the throat center and ears which give and receive sound, and the lungs and joints. The emotions associated with the ether element are grief for temporal relationships and things, or longing, caused by our separation from our divine source.

Excessive grief is a downward and outward movement toward the elements of earth, water, fire and air, for the world, people, things and realities that are transitory. Longing is an upward and inward movement which yearns for truth, spirituality, eternal love and divine union. When we are in grief, the present moment is wasted looking backward into what no longer exists and what is now only in the imagination. Mid–life can become a negative experience when women cling to the past. Perhaps children have grown, and there is neither career, husband or purpose to fill the vacuum. Grief becomes fixated on what was in the past, for things that have gone, instead of being directed toward the present, the inner life and spirituality. Grief is usually supported with fear, attachment, anger and greed as the individual blames God, the universe and the realities of life for not letting things be like they want or remain as they were.

Naturopathic purification creates space and relieves the system. Herbs offer superior nutrition for regeneration and achieving hormonal balance. Transformation unfolds as we are able to let go and allow our lives to unfold. We must turn this emotional grief for what we imagine is lost, upward and inward, toward spiritual yearning, prayer and meditation.

Lung, throat, voice, hearing and neck problems are associated with ether imbalances.

Positive ether elemental energy speaks, hears and knows truth and has the courage to experience the present reality at any given moment. Desire and longing are now directed upward and inward. The elements of earth, water, fire, and air no longer pull us into the world, but support our spiritual practice, which provides nourishment in such abundance that the radiant flow of love, happiness, joy, creativity and service is boundless.

Useful Bach flower remedies are: *Star of Bethlehem* gives comfort, *Mustard* relieves depression, *Gorse* uplifts hopelessness, *Gentian* neutralizes our attraction for negativity. *Nat. Mur.* or *Ignacia* homeopathic remedies help to relieve grief.

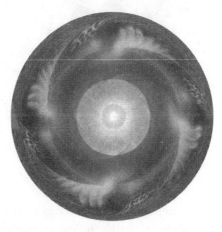
# BROW & CROWN SPIRITUAL CENTERS

## CONTENTMENT AND SPIRITUALITY
### SUPREME LONELINESS – DEATH IS IMAGINED AS AN END NOT A BEGINNING

The Brow and Crown chakras reside in the pituitary and pineal glands in the brain, and are beyond the elemental energies of earth, water, fire, air and ether. They contain subtle aspects of all the elements and their functions affect the elements.

While these higher centers cannot be considered emotional, they reflect the masculine and feminine energies within our bodies and throughout the cosmos. In Chinese philosophy the pituitary Brow center is considered to be the Dragon feminine force that manifests ideas and goals in the world, or that concentrates inwardly to become receptive to spirituality. The pineal Crown is considered to be the Tiger masculine force that fertilizes the feminine and nature with divine guidance and bliss.

Creative potential is all around us, yet many women do not know what to do with themselves and their lives. Instead of looking inward for guidance and giving willing service in whatever circumstances they find themselves, their inner world becomes full of negativity, complaining, deprivation, frustration and emptiness.

Spirituality is our natural inclination toward love, toward our Creator and toward divine union. This is as natural as a plant in its organic unfolding toward the sun. We need to let spirituality flower, bear fruit and produce seeds in our elder years of experience and wisdom. We need to nourish our spirituality and develop our inner life, so that conscious awareness is on the spiritual life, not on the physical.

Through surrender, acceptance, letting go and allowing ourselves to age naturally and gracefully with love and gratitude, we are awakened to our divine nature as we prepare ourselves to die consciously. By cooperating with the process we allow ourselves to be refined, tempered, sharpened, honed and shaped for our journey out of our body to our birth into the realm of spirit. Prepare for this transition by seeking spiritual teachers, living a simple and meaningful life and practicing meditation and prayer.

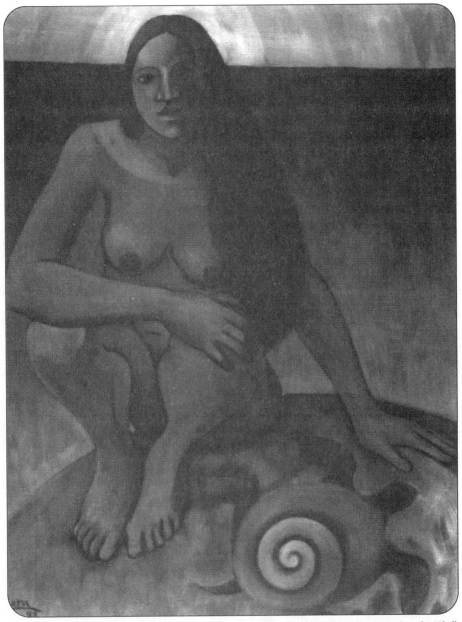

*Emerging from her Shell*

# HOMEOPATHIC EMOTIONAL BALANCING

These homeopathic remedies are recommended to relieve the excessive emotional states that may manifest in different personalities. Most homeopathic remedies can be purchased in low potencies up to 30x, in health food stores. Follow the directions on the bottle for the daily dose. We recommend consulting a homeopathic doctor for extreme emotional states.

*Apis Mellifica:* Apathy, indifference; unconsciousness; awkward; drops things; sudden cries or screams; jealous, fearful, angry, easily vexed and grief stricken; fidgety; whining; tearful; hard to please; cannot concentrate mind.

*Arsenicum Album:* Intense restless anxiety; fears something terrible is going to happen; possessiveness; finds fault easily; weakness; chilly; symptoms worse at night.

*Cimicifuga Racemosa:* Great depression with a sense of failure in relationships and business, impending evil; sensation of an enveloping cloud; self injury; incessant talking; delirium tremens; amenorrhoea; head pains; a good remedy for dark–haired women.

*Hydrastis:* Depressed; desires death; constipation; headaches.

*Hamamelis Virginica:* Wants the "respect that is due" shown to her.

*Ignatia:* Frequent loud sighing and sobbing but feels worse when consoled; unreasonable anger followed by a headache; symptoms are brought on by emotional excess.

*Kali Phosphoricum:* Mental and physical depression due to excitement, overwork and worry; nervous; irritable, night terrors; shyness; despondent about business; hysteria; headaches.

*Lachesis:* Excitability, together with vivid imagination; attacks of anxiety at night followed by sadness in the morning; jealous, suspicious; believes people are conspiring against her.

*Mercurius:* Aggravated by everything; agitation; restlessness; unable to concentrate; hurried speech; sudden anger accompanied by an urge to do violence.

*Natrum Muriaticum:* Extreme anxiety about everything; anxious dreams; ill after emotional trauma; introverted and solitary; can't handle rejection; keeps emotions inside; can't stand heat.

*Nux Vomica:* Anger with violent temper and sudden destructive impulses; irritable and quarrelsome; can't bear contradiction; fussy over details; chilly; digestive disorders.

*Rhus Toxicodendron:* Listless and sad with thoughts of suicide; extreme restlessness; constantly changing position; cannot sleep at night, or even remain in bed.

*Sepia:* Indifferent, even to loved ones; aversion to work and family; irritable; easily offended; dreads solitude; very sad, weeping when talking about self and symptoms; miserly; indolent.

# Cosmic Sexuality

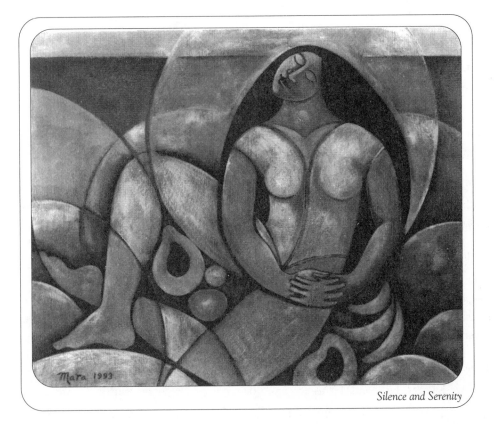

*Silence and Serenity*

Lifting the power of sexuality is one of the challenges of spirituality. Moving from personal sexuality to cosmic sexuality is an expansion of consciousness that not only improves physical sexuality but also utilizes the energies for spiritual growth. Instead of limiting sexuality to our personal experiences, programming and expectations, sexuality is transmuted to the divine dance of the male and female opposites of the universe. This macrocosmic dance is within us in microcosmic form. The sacred marriage of masculine and feminine within us helps us attain an integration of opposites that nourishes our wisdom and our spirituality.

Our sexuality is formed from both universal and parental energies from the earliest beginnings of our existence. It is shaped by the karmic patterning that draws us to our particular parents, by our conception within their sexual and spiritual experience, by our development in our mothers' wombs, by our birth and by our family atmosphere. From this conscious and unconscious content, our longings, our desires, our fears, our expectations and our sexual relationships with men and women manifest to help us seek balance, healing and completion. Our sexual experiences mirror the cosmic forces of masculine and feminine in the universe.

In our families we learn that worldly love can be associated with pain, rejection, shame, guilt, and dissatisfaction. Natural instincts toward love and affection may become inhibited or manipulative and cause us to move further and further away from our emotional truth. Some of us may have experienced sexual abuse during childhood, which will distort all our attempts at friendships or relationships. Others may emerge from their family cocoon completely innocent and unprepared for life, and suffer hard knocks as the world teaches them through experience. Others may ease slowly out of their family nest, without fuss or excitement, supported by family and friends, and move through their destiny as though they were sleepwalking. Undoubtedly there are women who are fully realized and fulfilled in this area of life, but all mid–life women have the opportunity to expand beyond personal sexuality into cosmic sexuality and the divine feminine. If we are unbalanced, we may attract a difficult relationship to help us learn.

It is generally recognized that we repeat experiences over and over again as we recreate dysfunctional patterns that are more familiar than the love, peace and harmony that we long for. We become attracted again and again to partners who prove that our distorted view of the universe is true. We armor ourselves against giving and receiving. We long for love, but we do everything possible to make sure that we do not find it. We pretend that we don't care about love and fashion our lives from solitude and compromise. We make excuses and weep silently at the loneliness we must endure without life partners. We marry for many reasons other than because we have truly found a harmonious friend, lover, mate or companion. We divorce out of desperation because the suffering of loneliness is better than the suffering of abuse or neglect. And yet, most women still have fantasies, dreams and longings for an ideal mate, a perfect love that wants to know us, honor us, respect us and share life with us. By the time we reach mid–life many of us have experienced the unhappy result of our dreams and our fantasies. We are ready to move on to something more real.

If we have to be alone, let us celebrate being alone. If we are with a partner let's do the work both individually and together to establish clear and true communication, with respect for our differences. If we have attained a balance of the masculine and feminine energies within us, we can more happily achieve and enjoy a relationship with a partner, or with our solitude.

During childhood we idealized and worshiped our parents, even if they were dysfunctional. They represented the masculine and feminine of our universe and we were dependent on them. Quickly we learned to interact with their reality as we fashioned our behavior to please, to rebel, to hide, to hate, to manipulate, to get what we wanted, to fear and to love. This adjustment shaped our being and slowly we became a part of that reality, acting out the undercurrents of unspoken truth. Whether we were lovingly prepared to leave our parents and our home, ran away, were afraid to leave, or whether it just happened naturally and easily, we met the forces of the universal masculine and feminine as our teachers until we were able to accept personal responsibility, achieve healing and restore harmony to our emotional lives.

It is only natural that we blame our parents, our boyfriends, our lovers and our mates for past wrongs, but as we reach the age of wisdom, we hopefully realize that we have to stop blaming. It is the time to change ourselves, to release, let go, forgive and recover our essential selves that exist beyond these dysfunctional patterns.

Sexuality is a focus and a forum for the acting out of our masculine and feminine distortions. Perhaps we were passive as young girls and succumbed without resistance to any male that chose to dominate us. Perhaps we were aggressive and enjoyed humiliating and teasing men. Perhaps we chose a provider and protector who made life safe for us. Perhaps we turned our back on men and chose artistic endeavors, academia, business or other women. Whatever role we chose we can be sure that it was shaped in reaction to our experiences during the early years of our lives. We seek our opposite. We seek the unknown. We seek passion, stimulation and companionship. We can remain unconscious, act out our male/female power struggles, achieve balance in relationship, or reach a place of hopelessness where we finally stop the externalization of desire and emotion and seek the integration of these energies within our beings.

Were we aware of our sexuality as young girls or was it a shock when we suddenly began to bleed? Did we hide this menarche, this flow of blood, or was it celebrated? How did our mother, sisters and friends react to this change? Did we have pain or other problems associated with our periods, puberty and early sexuality? In my generation and within my family and circle of friends we never talked about anything sexual. I never knew what periods were until I had one. I didn't know how babies were born until I was nearly seventeen. This innocent, ignorant time has vanished. Instead of rebelling against repression, young people today are media brainwashed into obsessive and seductive sexuality, glamour, clothes and makeup. For a time women experienced greater freedom due to tampons, the Pill and IUD's, and lived out a free sexuality without fear of pregnancy. But now, almost in response to increased promiscuity, sexuality has become associated with the deadly AIDS disease that fills us with renewed fear and caution for our sexual choices.

What was our first sexual experience like? Perhaps we gave in to peer pressure and lost our virginity in the back seat of a car with someone we hardly knew or cared about because we did not know how to say no. Perhaps we waited so long for our ideal mate that we missed more realistic opportunities. Perhaps we teased and petted so much that we lost the ability to relate to truth. Perhaps we exuded sexuality to attract and marry our mate and then retreated into indifference. Perhaps we were so passive and our mate so dominating that even after many years of marriage we had not yet expressed our authentic sexuality.

When we lost our virginity and were penetrated by a male partner, our mates helped us to learn about ourselves. Our sexual seeking had a greater truth behind it, that of attraction to our opposite. After years of sexual life experience women come to menopause older, wiser and richer. It is a time of change. Whereas at menarche our seeking was directed outward toward the male species, now we have the opportunity to penetrate ourselves and explore our feminine through our masculine. We have to become both male and female and learn how to integrate these two primal energies within ourselves, in our relationships and in our lives.

During teenage years our fathers may have started pushing us away because they became affected by our sexuality, or perhaps they died or left, depriving us of masculine energy and leaving us feeling unloved and unwanted. Perhaps our mothers' attitude of repressed sexuality was passed on to us, and we were made to feel ashamed of our monthly flow, our budding breasts and our unfoldment as a fertile young woman. Perhaps we watched other, more pretty and confident girls accept dating easily and naturally, while we were left out, unwanted and unpopular. Perhaps we were poor and had to work or take care of our family and missed the fun of youth. There are so many possibilities for the unfulfilled hunger of youth to seek, find and act out love needs, ideals and fantasies by claiming our sexual power. While these early experiences could have made us either more confident or taken our confidence away, they certainly helped us to learn about the world and the elemental dance of duality.

Our culture encourages us to marry, to settle down, to raise a family and to fulfill our roles as lover, wife and mother. These pressures force us into decisions that are not necessarily grounded in wisdom or clarity and we suffer the consequences. Even though we feel we could not have done anything other than what we did, we may emerge with a sense of failure and frustration, feeling that the world did not support our dreams of love and harmony. This awakening is often more than we can bear, and depression, despair and grief may overtake us.

Our roles as mothers encompass many experiences. Our children appear in our lives not only as responsibilities, but as teachers and as loving support. Although we have to sacrifice much to raise them and care for them, their sweet faces and loving eyes can nourish and support us through difficult times. Women both long for and resist motherhood. By the time women reach mid–life, mothers who have brought children into the world have nearly completed their responsibilities. Others who have not raised children may be mourning the fact that they never had this experience. Whatever the situation, it is time to open. We must let this natural aspect of femininity flow without resistance into all that we do. We can nourish the world from our essence and leave it richer for our presence here. We can become the Divine Mother.

When the honeymoon is over and married life begins to drain all our energies, sexuality often goes underground. The frustrations of being a wife and homemaker in today's world revolve around cultural perfection standards, materialism and increasing needs for women to combine family and careers. The stress and pressure are enormous. We manifest as many–armed–goddesses who run from duty to duty, keeping up and keeping everything together, performing haphazardly a multitude of outward activities. There are rare opportunities to balance these activities with stillness, deep feeling, and interior attention. During this time sexual experiences also diminish due to exhaustion, lack of time, unexpressed anger and lack of communication. To turn the tide on this culture–driven frenzy requires great determination and strength, but if we do not do it we end up as victims of our cultural disease. By the time we reach menopause we may be depleted, exhausted and disenchanted. We may have attained all our goals and still feel empty, or we may feel we are failures because our dreams of success have not come true. Whatever the situation, we have lost our enthusiasm for the 'carrots' of life. When we turn our attention within to reclaim our essence, the landscape seems like an empty, barren wasteland. We now yearn for something real, something pure, and something that is truth. We long for our lost selves that we have used up. We long for all that we wanted to do and did not, or could not, do. We mourn our mistakes, our wrong choices and our missed opportunities. This grief is a necessary part of our awakening, but we must not stay here. We must shake off the mourning for what never was or what could have been, and move on.

Our sexuality goes through changes during mid–life. In the past this time has been referred to as the 'mid-life crisis.' Whatever the individual story, women begin to make waves. As deeper

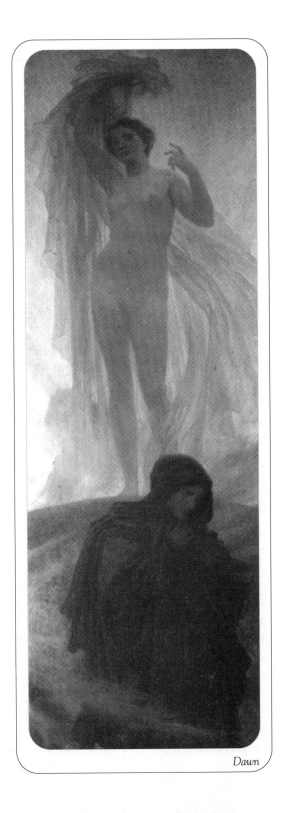

Dawn

levels of truth surface and the process of integration takes place, women who have been frigid, repressed or uninterested suddenly awaken to profoundly erotic passions. They may take lovers, leave mates, go on adventures and explore the outer world from a new ground of confidence and integration. Ideally they fall in love with all of life and begin to explore inner landscapes where boundaries and limitations dissolve. Sexuality loses its power over us if we transform to our next level of emergence, cosmic spirituality and universal wisdom. Our masculine and feminine unite within our being to bring peace, contentment, fulfillment and acceptance. We learn to make the most out of our situation, and above all we experience the unconditional love of true friendship. We no longer sacrifice our essence, our truth and our values in order to possess a sexual partner.

Some women hang on to sexuality as if it defined their existence. Money, resources, time, energy, interest and purpose are all devoted to looking young and being attractive. Women choose cosmetic surgery and spend fortunes on makeup and hair care. The games of glamour, seduction and relationships fill their world. If we allow ourselves to surrender to each different cycle of our lives with grace, intelligence and wisdom, we will manifest beauty at each stage. If we try to hang on to one stage and refuse to grow, we will miss our potential life experience.

Sexual addictions can manifest if there is enormous resistance to releasing, completing and integrating emotional wounds. Perversion may plague women or they may require psychiatric help or incarceration in a mental home. Whatever is not dealt with inwardly will manifest outwardly. What we refuse to face will meet us.

Internally we have to face the various aspects of our positive and negative sexuality. We have to look at all aspects of our feminine: the prostitute, the bitch, the cute little girl who refuses to grow up, the pleaser, the martyr, and the old hag, as well as the lover, the friend and the partner. Our ideal imaginary lover within us may suddenly manifest, either outwardly as a lover who may tear our life apart, or inwardly in fantasies that take us away from the reality of our present life. Both situations are avoidance of our spiritual selves that seek to transform, grow and prepare us for higher levels of consciousness. After menopause women are also free of fear of pregnancy and no longer have to use birth control devices or drugs.

Those who are in a love relationship may find that sexuality is better than ever, physically, sexually, emotionally, mentally and spiritually, when we are fully ourselves, relaxed within our being, complete and fulfilled. Now we can appreciate our partners and experience love more deeply. We are more free to express our sexuality, and the sense of companionship is rich and fulfilling. Menopause increases and deepens sexuality in whatever realms women wish to explore.

Divine love, the sacred marriage, and inner union are all concepts for states of being that defy description. Because outer sexuality seems so exciting, sensual and attractive, we cannot imagine how we could ever be satisfied with more subtle inner states, but the exquisite, light–filled bliss of these states of consciousness offer lasting happiness without all the difficulties of dealing with others' moods, needs and shortcomings. We find we no longer need a partner to feel the grace of love, longing and desire. All of it happens within us and it is utterly satisfying. We become whole in body, mind and spirit, whether we are in a love partnership or not. When we attain spiritual wholeness this enhances any relationship we have in our lives, especially our relationship with ourselves.

# Mental Winnowing

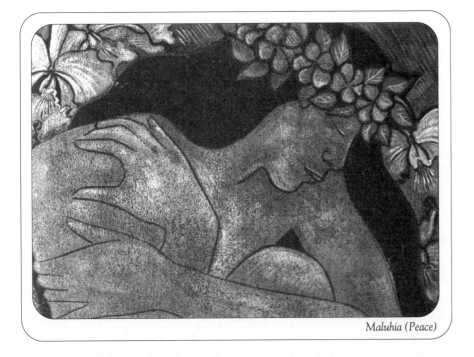

Maluhia (Peace)

Separating cultural myths and truths through our discriminating processes helps us attain our authentic reality, a ground of being that is formed from our instincts, our feelings, our experiences, our knowledge and our wisdom. When we function from this authentic base we remain in touch with truth and allow it to blossom in every aspect of our lives.

We come to mid–life during our maturity, when we are fully formed in the eyes of the world, and yet most of us still hold our wounds, our longings and our potential in internal chaos. Mature on the outside, we live like infants, children or teenagers in our emotional lives, acting out our confusion, our defenses and our unbalanced desires. Somehow life has passed us by and we have never matured fully. Perhaps we have been too busy. We may have allowed ourselves to be driven by the outer world. We may not be able to keep down our unconscious shadow and yet we still deny its effect on our lives. Whatever the reason for this accumulated negative content, mid–life comes during the surfacing of the shadow. The roots and stems of our thoughts, feelings and actions have been growing about forty years, and mid–life is the time of our harvest. We may have sown roses, but we also may have sown strong and lusty thistles among them that cause us great suffering.

Our inner life is like a garden and when our thoughts, needs, desires, actions and feelings have grown haphazardly, there is a random harvest. The relentless driving energy required to keep our daily lives together has forced us to ignore the more subtle calls from our undeveloped inner being. Menopause comes at a time when we must look clearly at the truth of our lives and prune all that does not belong to our essence. We have to live out the promise of the roots of our lives, whether good or difficult, happy or sad. So, let us take the time to sift through our minds and our hearts. Let us dig out the roots of the thorny bushes and prickly thistles, and give our energy to the thoughts and feelings that will create the lives that we want for ourselves. When we were young we did not have the maturity and leisure for such conscious discrimination. Now we must make time to do this work, so that we can jettison our heavy baggage and fly freely upward to our highest destiny.

As we explore the myths and truths of aging in the coming pages, each section will give examples of positive and negative mental mantras – repetitive thoughts that we repeat again and again, which create and define our reality. These examples not only help us to sift through and recognize any negative thought forms that are influencing our unfolding reality, but they also provide us with positive alternatives.

## AGING MYTHS

In this youth–oriented culture our aging myths teach us to be ashamed of physical fading. Desperate fears of loneliness, of being unwanted, useless, invisible and ugly keep us focused on superficial appearances rather than on what is spiritual, creative and authentically, radiantly beautiful within us. Women spend their resources of time, energy and money on clothes, jewelry, makeup, hair treatments and face–lifts because they are conditioned to believe glamour, seductiveness, youth and physical perfection are beauty. Impossible ideals leave women in a constant state of frustration at their imperfections and vulnerable before the judgment of other's eyes and minds. Women sustain this illusion through cooperation with these myths.

Aging has become synonymous with negativity. Because we fear that we will be weak, sick, poor, unwanted or unattractive, we do not imagine that our elder years can be a time of happiness or fulfillment. It is as though some essential core of strength has been lost, and aging has become identified with loss and dependence. If we seek to enjoy the fruits of our elder years, we have to nourish the roots that will sustain them – creativity, independence, good health, exercise, moderate living habits and simple pleasures.

Elderly aborigine women were noble, productive, active, valued and happy in old age, within their own culture. Because other primitives believed that women would die when they stopped their period, women continued to bleed past eighty years. Native cultures valued women's retreats during the monthly cycle because they offered rest, time for introspection and spiritual and feminine nourishment. Ancient peoples celebrated women's passage beyond the fertility cycle to the honored circle of the crone, the wise woman and the elder. Today we have to lift ourselves out of the time frame and context of our culture to free ourselves from the negative myths and illusions that surround our cycles and menopause. Because we have no positive cultural definition as in ancient times, we have the freedom to explore the challenge of our own uniquely individual creative change of life.

We also have to examine what we think of as beautiful. Once we free beauty from time, fashion, glamour, projections, ideals, comparisons and limitation, we find beauty everywhere, in every age, culture, race, body type and personality. We must reexamine youth culture obsessions with slimness, muscle tone, smooth facial skin and superficial personalities, and learn to appreciate the beauty of spirit and experience, the charm of wrinkles, white and silver hair, fuller body shapes and authentic personalities that radiate wisdom, strength, courage, creativity and love. Look for elderly people who radiate beauty from within, who are happy and who enjoy their lives, and let them inspire you. As menopausal women we have to be living examples of our uniquely personal beauty, our creative life and our joyful potential.

Negative aging mantras for aging may be: I am dying, fading away, becoming wrinkled, unattractive and decrepit. I must do everything I can to stay young. I cannot allow myself to become old because no one will want me. I cannot be myself.

## AGING TRUTHS

An authentic woman is beautiful from her core, from her spirit and from the love and creativity that manifests in her relationship with her family, the community, the world and her personal spiritual life. True beauty shines out. The light and radiance of spirituality inspires magnetic attraction. Old age is beautiful. Remember as children how we loved older people, yet our culture discards them. Some older women give up on life. Others who are wise and wonderful are sought out by many, are never alone and are greatly loved, valued and appreciated. We can blame and fear the world and our old age, but if we make something of ourselves, these fears need never manifest.

As a child I was greatly inspired by my favorite comic strip, Mary Worth, a beautiful, serene elderly woman who was sought after by friends and relatives who wanted her to be part of their lives. She went from situation to situation, contributing support, love, wisdom and caring. Her example provided me with a very positive role model for an elderly person. Old age does not necessarily mean that others will take care of us and we will offer nothing. There are many cultures that value their elders, storytellers, teachers, medicine and wise women, those that hold and share the knowledge with coming generations. When elders are valued by society they live fulfilled lives, and the community benefits greatly from their contribution.

We have to redefine aging. We have to stop ourselves from indulging in fears that we will become an old hag and be ugly, decrepit and shriveled up, or our worst fears about aging will manifest. Age is not pathetic. We have a deep potential ahead. We need to set an example and seed our culture with the potential of new roles, new possibilities and new power. The Celtic myths tell of the three cycles of the female: the virgin, the mother and the crone. The virgin is the flower, the mother the fruit and the crone the seed that regenerates the community and the world with the wisdom gathered through her lifetime. The seed contains the full pattern for the future, and the flower and the fruit are contained in the seed. The virgin and the wife and mother are inspired, supported and guided by the feminine elders who are content, serene and wise in their roles. The elders are happy because their contribution to the raising of the young is valued and their support of the mothers during their years of responsibility is appreciated. The wise woman contributes to and is a valuable part of everyone's lives, and the community gains by the circle of love and wisdom that flows through the three cycles of womanhood.

Menopausal women are free to be themselves, to speak and live the truth, to be outrageous and break all bounds when they are no longer restricted by the roles of virgin, wife and mother. Women fear invisibility and loss of sexual glamour, but these can be considered gifts instead of problems. Now we can move as we wish, and no one knows or guesses what we are doing or contributing, or how full we are within our being. This is a blessing in disguise. If we perceive this change as neglect, rejection or abandonment, we lose an opportunity to discover and enjoy a valuable part of our menopausal experience.

Now is the time we can make a difference, because we are free from the responsibilities of child–rearing and family life. Now we have time for creativity, to teach and guide the young, to support worthwhile projects and influence the future of our world. Because our time is more our own than it has ever been, we can choose to use it to make our dreams come true, both for ourselves and for those we love, in the service of both our inner and outer worlds. If we can truly awaken to what an exciting time it is, we will be able to take full advantage of the creative opportunity of mid–life.

Positive aging mantras might be: Now I know that beauty is within and that it shines out. If there are those who see only my aging, that is their problem. Those that love and value me, do so because of who I truly am. I love my aging. My wrinkles tell the story of my love and my survival. I love my silver hair that is like a crown on my head. I look at the young women around me and I am grateful that I have arrived at this time of fulfillment and that I am happy, at peace and content. I love to share my wisdom and experience with those around me.

## SEXUAL MYTHS

We are so conditioned to equate success with being sexually desirable that the fears of not being attractive, of not being desired by men, of loss of romance, of being alone, of losing a life partner cause shame as well as inhibition of other significant relationship values. Friendship and partnership is devalued when the prime relationship is seductive. Women need to value themselves beyond their sexual roles and challenge men to honor them. When women feel more attractive and more valuable within themselves they exude the strength and confidence that will influence the men in their lives as well as their culture.

Negative sexual mantras might be: My sexuality is increasing within me just when I am becoming less attractive. I have to accept any relationship I can get. I should consider myself lucky to have a sexual partner. I'll do anything to keep this man in my life. I don't want to be alone. Others will look at me and feel sorry for me if I am on my own. Now that I am not fertile I feel barren. I feel as if I have no sexual value. I am experiencing menopause and men don't like that. I'm afraid to tell my partner I am in menopause. I am embarassed that my body is changing and aging. I don't want my lover to see my wrinkles and the lack of tone in my body so I always turn off the lights. I am ashamed of my body now and that affects my love making.

## SEXUAL TRUTHS

Surface attraction without the richness of inner feelings cannot compare to a relationship of depth and communion that brings forth deep happiness because it is fed by inner spiritual springs. Sacred sexuality that is not driven only by hormones and lust is to be greatly valued, as are vulnerability and intimacy with a true partner/friend where love is born of consciousness and awareness, not from need, desire and projection. It is also important to be able to enjoy being alone until a partner of value comes along. And if no one comes, the inner marriage and one's relationship to divine love will nourish and uplift life energies and leave one satisfied with all of life. True happiness comes from an inward completeness of being. Relationships should be based on sharing and caring friendships, not on need. The truth is that we have more to offer during our menopausal years, not less. We are nourished internally and experience contentment.

Positive sexual mantras might be: I have become so much greater than my sexuality. I value myself and don't need anyone else to validate my existence. If I attract a partner, great, I will enjoy that, and if not, I am very happy on my own. I get to do what women cannot do when they are enmeshed in relationships. Many women long for the privacy and freedom that I have. I consider myself very fortunate. I am in love with all of life and experience love in many different dimensions of my inner and outer life. My capacity for love has increased. When I am with a partner it is better than it has ever been before. I realize now that I am much more than just my body. The joy I experience in my love relationship now is greater than ever before.

## MENTAL MYTHS

We believe that as we age memory and concentration will become impaired and that we will become out–of–date, old–fashioned. We fear that we won't be able to keep up, that we won't be able to communicate and that people won't want to talk to us. Through negativity and fear we criticize and condemn those around us and complain about what the world is coming to instead of staying vital and alive. If we haven't taken care of our health we may suffer from poor memory and our senses may become impaired. Our energy does change as we get older and we do move to a slower beat, but that measured beat can draw the rushing, active, driven young into it to give them peace. There is no excuse for opting out. We create what we become, and we suffer the consequences or enjoy the harvest. There is also a fear of Alzheimers, of losing control.

Negative mental mantras might be: I can't keep up with the world. All the good things are gone. Things aren't what they used to be. I don't want to be part of what is happening today. I can't make all these new fangled contraptions work – buttons and wires and computers, it's all too confusing. I'm left out and left behind. I already feel dead.

## MENTAL TRUTHS

The truth is that the 'knowing' of our elder years is wisdom, not the sharp memory that astounds everyone with quickness, memory and agility when we are young. Wisdom is slower, more intuitive, more reflective. Often elders take a long time to answer a question, as they sift through different layers of truth. Many times the answer may be a question, or a joke that shocks or stimulates the questioner into making changes in their life. We may fear a lack of mental ability but the truth is that we may have a wider mental capacity that is of far greater value than anything we achieved mentally in our younger days. This mental ability may not be so goal- or profit-oriented, but it is not to be devalued for that reason.

As elders we have the opportunity to see truth and know truth, not to run from it. As survivors we have years of experience behind us. We have learned the ropes and can play the game. We may no longer have to work for a living. We may now have resources and funds at our disposal. Now it is time to develop our higher mind and our creativity. Opportunity abounds. Freedom awaits us. We can become a storyteller, a writer, an artist or a healer. If we can let go of what always stopped us from doing what we wanted when we were young, we can do it now. That is the gift of our elder years. Take it. Don't let this opportunity go by.

Positive mental mantras might be: My mind works better than it ever has, because it is enriched by experience, wisdom and integration. I am able to see farther than the impatient young people around me, and I can caution and guide them in wise decisions. My mind is more easily uplifted by my inner life and less attracted to temporal things around me. It is also less affected by the thoughts and actions of those around me. My mind is now a vehicle for my essence. Instead of running me, I use and direct my mind to achieve my highest purpose.

## FAMILY MYTHS

In our culture the concept of the extended family has been discarded. Young people leave home to live alone or with strangers their own age. Newly married couples struggle to pay rent or buy a home and all the material things they need, and young parents are isolated with their children. Life is lived on the run. There is never enough time, never enough money and never enough of yourself to go around. The flight from parents, grandparents, uncles and aunts may provide the opportunity to escape domination, 'do your own thing' and experience a degree of freedom. However, the loss of companionship, sharing of and household duties and financial support has contributed to our cultural obsession with money and material things. This takes our attention away from valuing the simple pleasures of family relationships and a quiet home life. With our actions we are running away from intimate and loving relationships, and transforming our lives into material symbols and possessions that can never satisfy us. In our old age we can become isolated within our independent material world and restricted by our hardened heart that had to shut down while we worked and strived to create our personal material world. Our lives have become so individual that we find it harder and harder to fit in with other people, even if they are our own relatives. We don't want to adjust to other people. We want our own space. When I am in India, people always ask me why I want to live alone. They say they would feel too isolated. They do not want quiet or space because they enjoy the sounds of other members of the family. They want to feel that they are surrounded and protected by their family and that someone will always be there. I explain to them that there are many benefits to living alone. Whatever our situation, whether alone or with others, we can make the most out of the opportunity.

Negative family mantras might be: My children don't want me anymore. I'm a nuisance. They are so noisy, I can't be around them. I don't understand the new generation. They just want to put me away. I don't know how to talk to them. I'll be a burden on them. I'll be weak and ill and in pain and dependent on them. They only want my money. They can't wait for me to die.

## FAMILY TRUTHS

If we rejoice in family roles, whether they be wife, mother, godmother, grandmother, great grandmother, sister, aunt or cousin, relatives will want us to be part of their lives. They will long for our visits and come to see us. Help them. Listen to them. Be sincerely interested in what is happening to them. Join them for major events in their lives – graduations, weddings, showers and holidays. Have adventures together. Take someone on a trip. Make a dream come true. Join in their lives. Open up to their music, books, activities and friends. Learn from them. Be there with them in their lives. Enjoy them. Let them be who they are. Share who you are. Be a role model for others. We can discover what family means to us and have the courage to love and share and laugh and cry and be fully human. For some the family may extend outward to communities or groups that share a common purpose, and for others the entire human race. Wherever and whatever family is, it is important to realize that loving companionship enriches our lives. The giving and receiving of love and caring is an essential function of human life that keeps us fully human and alive.

Positive family mantras might be: Now that I am older and my life is more peaceful I have more time to enjoy all the family and social relationships in my life. Because I am happy and fulfilled within myself I enjoy giving to others. My life has become rich in love. I also feel that everyone is my family and I look for opportunities to be of service wherever and whenever I can. As I grow older I enjoy making my life more simple. I enjoy giving away what I no longer want or need for myself. Things or events used to be the cause of any happiness. Now I am just happy within myself. It is love, the giving and receiving love in every form, that is of value to me now. I don't want to hold on to everything and have it distributed after my death. I enjoy giving. It makes me happy to watch people enjoy what I give.

## SOCIAL MYTHS

Our culture sees retirement and old age as an ending. Life experience is not valued. Instead of gaining status in old age we are devalued. Instead of being included we are excluded. When society does not value or honor the elderly, except when they make some monumental achievement, and when retirement is an end, not a beginning, we feel that our life is over and that our elderly years are a wasteland. In African societies, when men complete their warrior phase they are welcomed into their elder status. When women complete their fertile phase they are honored as wise women and healers. They do not leave a phase of their life without being welcomed to their next level. There is never an end without a beginning.

Because our society does not place value on its older people other than what they may win for themselves through position, power, achievement or money, aging women often become negative and fearful. Energy is used in contracted, self–limiting projections that stop women from living out their positive dreams. It is important to open the heart center and to celebrate life by keeping the flow of loving, giving and receiving moving. We are alive, so let's be fully alive. We can contribute to society in many different ways. If something needs to be done, do it, however big or small. Keep the giving and receiving of love moving in all aspects of our lives. Let's be responsible for our roles in the universe, play those roles well and enjoy the performance.

Negative social mantras might be: I am a burden on society. I have saved for my retirement all my life; but now I don't know what to do with myself. I feel useless. I was a valuable person when I was working. Now I have nothing to do. I am useless. No one wants me. I have no purpose. I have so many years to waste in nothingness. I am bored. I hope I don't live much longer. No one will miss me when I go.

## SOCIAL TRUTHS

The truth is that as long as we feel as though we are a part of society there is work for us to do and a part to play in daily life. According to our attitude we can make this as positive as we choose. It is generally unknown that the Constitution of the United States of America was based on an Iroquois Indian treaty. All aspects of the treaty were incorporated into the Constitution except one requiring that all governing decisions be put before the Grandmothers, who were privileged to give the absolute yes or no based on whether they thought the decision honored life or not. The women elders were respected by those who wished to give the best to their society, because their communities believed they would make the best decision for all concerned. The fact that the founding fathers of America only left this out of the Constitution suggests that they deliberately decided not to incorporate the value of women's wisdom into government. At that time women were kept at home, dependent on men and not allowed to vote. As women, let us take back our role of wise counselor and decision maker for our society and stand straight and tall in the fullness and richness of our menopausal and elder years.

Positive social mantras might be: Now that I don't have to make a living I can do what I always wanted to do. I can work for a nonprofit organization, save the whales, help a president get elected, visit the dying, read to the blind, help my neighbor, baby-sit for a single mother or make meals for the homeless. I receive happiness by being of service to people, by helping out. I enjoy the time I have and it puts a song in my heart. People come over often to talk and visit. In my small way I contribute to a better world. I have surplus money to share so I can help my family, my friends, contribute to worthwhile causes, and make good things happen in this world.

## WORK MYTHS

There are work myths instilled in us from early childhood that make us feel ashamed if we are not working. We learn that we are judged by the work that we do and how much we are paid for it. Menial workers or poor people are not valued; they are usually abused and underpaid. Yet some doctors and lawyers, who may not be good at their job, or even honest, make a lot of money and have a high status in our society. Success is equated with a good job and a big salary, not with character values, such as integrity, honesty and loyalty, which are often sacrificed to the gods of power and success. The American dream is built on getting ahead, producing and winning, even at the expense of others. Often personal talents, gifts and dreams are ignored and put off, because people feel they cannot do the work they love. They feel obligated to train and work at a job that society will respect and that will provide a good living. Parents force their offspring to train at jobs or follow in their footsteps. The children are not allowed to follow their natural inclinations or to develop their own talents, and their lives are lived to please their parents.

The reality in our society is that many women are forced to work at positions beneath their level of expertise, receive lower salaries than men, or become like men in order to succeed. They sacrifice much to make their own money and enjoy independence. They may not believe that they could make a living being themselves and doing what they love. On the other hand, work can become synonymous with freedom and reflect personal creative choices. Work affects menopause if it decreases or limits our choices. Women often hang onto jobs that offer health insurance and pension plans, rather than take a leap and do something they want to do, because they want to make sure they will be taken care of.

Negative work mantras might be: I am so afraid of losing my job, my money and my independence that I will do anything to keep them. I wouldn't know what to do if I lost my job. I have to keep looking young, so they won't lay me off. They don't want old employees. They want me to retire, but I want to keep working. I am afraid to take time off even when I am sick. Now that I'm retired I'm useless and don't know what to do with myself every day. I always looked forward to retirement and now that it is here, I don't know what to do with myself. I got a job in the five and dime just for something to do, so I could be out in the world and see people and feel like I am doing something. I don't work as well as I used to. I can't remember things. I feel like the world is passing me by. I'm not contributing anything. My whole life has passed by and I never got to do what I wanted to. I know I was capable of so much more. Why did I keep putting my dreams aside?

## WORK TRUTHS

We must ask ourselves what work means to us. We must follow our hearts, our creativity and our instincts, and do work that we love. Work is such a big part of our lives. When our lives and hearts become entwined in our work, work becomes a vehicle for love. Higher states of consciousness can also enlighten and uplift any type of work or service if there is not a particular call to a special kind of work. We must explore our relationship to work and seek new frontiers of expression and unfoldment.

Positive work mantras might be: I always had to work everyday at a job I didn't like, be there no matter what, and now I'm free and I can do the work I love. I work for less because I love to do this work, and when I'm not working I enjoy my home, my garden, and my hobbies. My life and my work have blended into one. I do part–time work at home. I volunteer for causes I believe in and work for nothing. I no longer need the position, the money or the power. I find happiness and satisfaction in what I do. This is the best time of my life.

## MEDICAL MYTHS

When doctors write in books that the ovary has failed, it sounds as if they believe that menopause is a disease instead of a change and growth process. In their reality our very hormones have become products, pills and drugs. The medical profession believes that most women are not capable of producing the correct balance of hormones. However, they do not consider the effect that contraceptive pills, other drugs, spermicides, IUD's, surgeries, diet, lifestyle or the poisons and pollutants of this world we live in, have had on our general health and on our hormones. The concept that a woman can live a natural life, have a healthy menopause and enjoy an even greater role in her elder years is something most doctors do not consider possible. Also, men often resent the independent power of the elder spiritual woman whose happiness is not dependent on being desired and valued by men. In the past, millions of women were tortured and murdered as witches so that men could take control of their wealth, their spiritual wisdom and their expertise as midwives and natural healers. Today, our present generation of menopausal women has the opportunity to become complete, whole, healthy and productive both during and after menopause and to take our place in the world as a positive, nurturing and wise force.

Most gynecologists and doctors only see ill, debilitated, frightened or helpless menopausal women in their consulting rooms, yet 80% of menopausal women have no major problems. The real problem lies in the fact that the doctors are conditioned both by their professional prejudices and by the experiences they have with their female patients. They are also affected by the modern business and media realities they do not believe that menopausal women can be healthy or enjoy their lives unless they are on hormone replacement therapy. These attitudes increase women's vulnerability and our dependence on doctors. Because women are not listened to, respected or treated in a holistic way, we are pressured into using drugs, having rush surgeries and treatments without being given time to think about the consequences or try alternatives. Unless a strong stand is taken to resist, many women end up mourning lost organs. Once we enter into the medical process it is difficult to break free.

This is not to say that modern medicine does not save lives or give service to humanity. The system itself, based as it is on profit and radical treatments, is to blame. True preventive education, instruction in healthy living, therapeutic treatments given in the early stages of development of conditions, together with cooperative communication by both doctors and patients, would lead us toward a compassionate medicine of the future.

In the hundreds of case histories I have taken over the years, a theme arises in almost every woman's history. Time and again women would talk to their doctor about something that was bothering them. Most often they were patronized, told it was only in their mind or that it was nonsense and given tranquilizers and pain pills. Only when the problem surfaced as a major life–threatening disease did the doctors recognize its reality, and take control with drug therapy, surgery, radiation and chemotherapy. They did not apologize for not listening for all those years. They did not take responsibility for all the years of pain, symptoms and malfunctions, or the eventual condition. Modern medical care is crisis care, not true healing. The present–day health system is a disease–oriented system.

Negative medical mantras might be: I am helpless. I don't know what to do. I can't deal with this because I'm not an expert. I have to turn myself completely over to my doctor and do everything that he says. I don't have the right to question his authority.

## MEDICAL TRUTHS

The truth is that like our breaths, heartbeats and days, the number of eggs in our ovaries are limited. We have a life before our periods start and we have a life afterward. Women need to penetrate the myth and illusion of modern medicine and see things as they are. Menopause is not a disease, but it has become a medical business because of the immense profits involved in giving millions of women hormone replacement therapy. Drug companies create advertising fads which purposefully prey on the fears of old age. We have the choice either to become a victim of their brainwashing or to live out our strength, truth and creativity. We do not have to succumb to their reality, which is based on prejudice, limited truth, profit seeking and manipulation. Our bodies and our lives belong to us as a gift from our Creator. Whatever choices we make, we are the ones who have to experience the consequences of any decision. Instead of giving ourselves over to someone else, we have to dive deep into our own wisdom and strength. There is a growing support system for those who seek to know themselves and to take responsibility for their body, emotions, mind and spirit. We need to ask for and allow ourselves to receive help.

The truth is that there are many healthy women enjoying their life before, during and after menopause. I ask you to take up the challenge of the creative mid–life. The truth is that many female problems could be avoided entirely by dealing with the small complaints as they appear, not suppressing them or denying them, by working with natural health practitioners, psychotherapists, herbalists, reflexologists, massage therapists, osteopaths and chiropractors. The dialogue with our bodies must be an active learning process experienced over many years so that a major crisis is not necessary to bring us back in touch with our bodies. If doctors do not listen with attention and respect, or explain truthfully what is happening, we have to make efforts to find different doctors. If our medical practitioners will not help us clear small symptoms as they occur, we must seek out alternative practitioners and natural health educators who will support our relationships with our holistic body–emotions–mind–spirit dynamic. We must take responsibility as early as possible so we won't become victims in the hands of modern medicine.

Positive medical mantras might be: I am my own healer. I take responsibility for creating my own health problems and for healing them. This does not mean that I do not seek advice or take treatments, but I discriminate consciously. I do not allow others to make my decisions for me. I will not allow others to pressure me. My wise woman within always makes the right choices. I do my best to live a healthy lifestyle. I enjoy taking care of my body and my health. I choose to use my money to pay for regular preventive care and massage instead of paying high premiums for disease care. I choose a catastrophe insurance for emergencies but I take my own health care as my personal responsibility.

## CREATIVE MYTHS

In this material and youth oriented culture creativity has become associated with youth, sexuality, confidence, prestige training at status schools, technical expertise, popular success, professionalism and products. We idolize professional artists, musicians, actors and actresses and designers, instead of developing these abilities in our own lives. Women are seen as creative when they produce products for the marketplace, but are devalued in their role as mothers and homemakers because these are not considered creative. It is ironic that when women become menopausal and are fully available for creativity, they are again devalued as infertile and made to feel that their creativity is over.

Negative creative myths are formed by materialism and commercialism. We have to free creativity from these fetters and return to the pure joy of creating something from raw materials. When we create, whatever we make does not need to be perfect, as if it were made by a machine. We need to let our gifts and talents develop naturally. We should develop skills by practicing and seeking teachers. The important thing is to enjoy creativity as a regular part of life. It is not something special or something that only artists do. Creativity is within each one of us, and it is up to us to awaken its flow. Primitive peoples make their own clothes, homes and utensils. Every member of their community is an artist who can create many different useful and beautiful crafts.

Negative creative mantras might be: my creative time is over. I can no longer make babies. My peers have all established themselves. It is too late for me. I always wanted to write a book, but never had time. I was always too busy raising my family. I don't have the training. What will people think. I am ashamed to let anyone see what I do. It is not good enough. What's the use? What would I do with what I make anyway? People would think I was crazy. I agonize over creativity. I get writer's block and sit for hours without being able to write a word. I always wanted to be creative, but now it's too late.

## CREATIVE TRUTHS

Authors like Isaac Dinesen and Hildegarde of Bingen started writing at about fifty years of age. Our best creativity comes when we have lived a full life and completed the process of integration. Women can now share their essence and their wisdom in mature creative works.

We must value ourselves as creative beings. We do not need the acceptance or approval of others to feel fulfilled in our creativity. We must learn to rejoice in the free, pure creativity of energy flowing through us every day into everything we touch and do. Our culture has materialized creativity into products. We buy things as if mere choice and purchase were creative acts. How many people create or decorate their own clothing and make things by hand, mixing their life energy with a raw material and making it part of their world? Traditionally women have surrounded themselves with creativity through cooking, gardening, decorating and crafts such as stitchery, basketry, quilting, weaving, jewelry and pottery – creating a uniquely personal world around themselves and their families. Creativity must be freed from judgment. It must spring freshly from our source as a celebration of our love, joy and enthusiasm for life. If we create purely from enthusiasm, time, practice and discrimination, the increasing skill will refine our work until we attain a natural mastery. Fear stops the flow of creativity. Doing what we love to do increases it. We must not hold back any longer. We must do what we have always longed to do. We must keep our lives in creative motion.

Positive creative mantras might be: I am creative because I want to be and because it flows naturally from me. I enjoy the process. I may try to get published at some point, but enjoying the creative process is the real goal. I enjoy creativity. It's something great that I do every day. Creativity is everywhere in my life. My garden, my herbs, my food, my relationships, my dress and my home are creative expressions of who I am. Now I can really be me. Creativity is my whole life. I can be outrageously myself – explore, have adventures and seek the highest in life – my spiritual creativity in my relationship with my inner life and the divine.

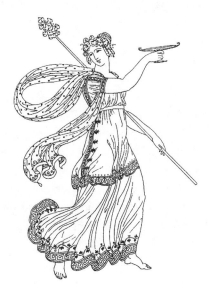

## SPIRITUAL MYTHS

We are taught from our early days that we need an intermediary between ourselves and the divine. We are discouraged from approaching God directly. We feel inhibited and turn our prayers into a long list of wants and needs. The personal, living relationship between ourselves and God may even be discouraged by the church. Life becomes far too busy and we pay lip service to an increasingly diminishing inner world. Our sexual, material world pulls us away from spirituality. Complicated lives make simplicity impossible. We are used up in the pursuit of success, and then, when we face illness and death, we wonder how our lives has passed us by so quickly. We realize as we approach our departure from this world that we are unprepared.

Negative spiritual mantras might be: I have never been a spiritual person – never had the time and now it is too late. I cannot live in the world, have a husband and kids and still be spiritual. I don't know how to pray and I don't know what meditation is. I feel out of place and unconnected spiritually. I am afraid, so I drink or watch TV all day, because I do not know what to do or where to go. I never could talk to the minister. Church doesn't make me feel spiritual. I feel spiritual in church but the feeling doesn't carry over into my daily life.

## SPIRITUAL TRUTHS

The truth is that spirituality is within us, waiting, longing for us to awaken to its presence, and make a living connection. It is not something outside of ourselves. Like everything else, it needs to be exercised and developed. If we long from our deepest seed soul for the flowering of spirituality, it will unfold. In the early stages of spirituality the experience is one of longing and seeking. Like the seed beneath the earth, our spiritual soul seeks the sun of the divine. It is also true that spirituality is a needed preparation for death. We know that we will leave this body and this world, and yet we live most of our lives pretending that we will be here forever. Most of our energy and life essence is spent either seeking pleasure and fulfillment from the world, or in working and taking care of duties and responsibilities.

During mid–life we can take the freedom that is now available and use it to awaken and explore the inner life and our spiritual dimensions. The journey can be wonderful. Take retreats. Go to sweat lodges. Learn meditation. Travel to India, Nepal or Japan to seek teachers and live in ashrams. We can also choose to go deeply and quietly within ourselves with a spiritual practice in our own homes, in our own community. Each person's movements of the soul are unique and each journey is made on the blank page of our personal destiny. Follow the longing. Let it take us within. Let it take us upward into spiritual life and downward into grounding. We must stretch the boundaries of our being. We are spiritual beings. We must discover what that means for ourselves.

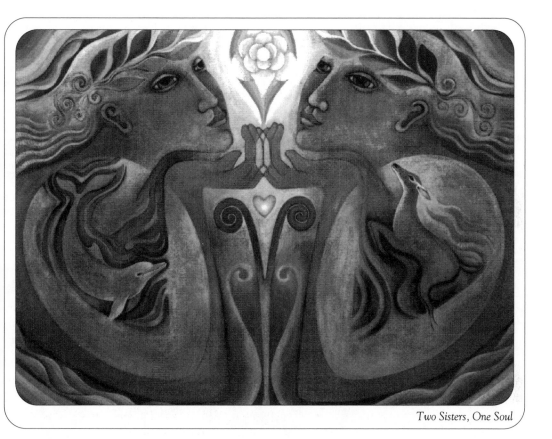

*Two Sisters, One Soul*

We have to develop an inner life both to sustain ourselves and also to become a source for what we give in relationship with the world. Ideally, as we evolve our inner and outer worlds will reflect each other. The richness of our inner lives, containing our strength, wisdom, perseverance, creativity, joy and contentment, will be reflected in loving companionship, based on consciousness, not co-dependence, desire or need. Women can feel the same sacredness of being whether alone or in the company of others. This sacredness can be with us in every cell of our bodies and in every aspect of our being. We can rejoice in our release and the return of our soul to the divine source at the time of physical death.

Positive spiritual mantras might be: Now that I have the time to explore and develop spirituality, I will go to church, study yoga, learn meditation, meet different teachers, take workshops and seminars, read books and enjoy exploring this part of life I never had time for before. Now that I am older I wake up early in the morning and know that this time is for prayer and meditation. I also see that spirituality is everywhere, in everything I do. I am preparing consciously for my death. I see that the release of my body opens up a new dimension of spirit. It is the time to make my connection and peace with my God and to go within and prepare. I see that menopause is a great preparation for this journey of my soul. I see that I was given the opportunity to let go, to complete, to integrate and discriminate. Because I am doing my work during my mid–life, I will be able to enjoy a rich harvest during my elder years.

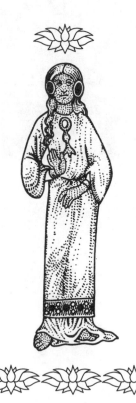

# Spiritual Transformation

*'We have to let go of life before it lets go of us.'*

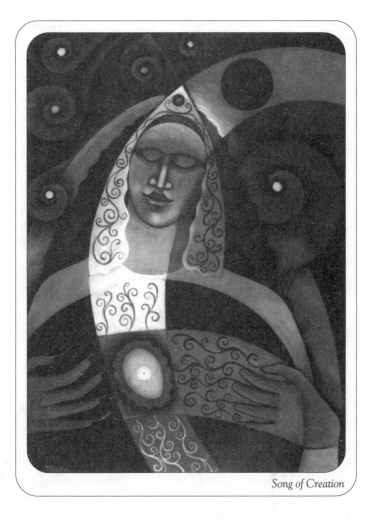

*Song of Creation*

    Dissolving into the divine can only be realized according to the level of surrender we are able to achieve. The self–death and the self–birth we experience during our mid–life change prepares us for our next transition, that of our self–death out of our body and this world into our self–birth in the realms of the spirit. Instead of agonizing through the process of dying we can learn to cooperate and turn our attention to what is emerging. We can work with and develop our inner lives, so that we can depart as clear and empty as when we came into this world. We celebrate birth into this world. We can learn to celebrate birth into the realms of spirit.

Menopause is a movement upwards. When we come into our forties and fifties the tide of procreative sexuality and outward energies begins to shift inward and upward. As our ovaries release our last eggs and our hormones change, the challenge and the opportunity to open our higher centers of consciousness become a reality we face every day, either consciously or unconsciously. If we cling to what is already passing away, we get stuck. Disease patterns and mental, emotional imbalances act out our refusal to move and change. But if we cooperate consciously with the process, the treasures that lie ahead will be greater than exploring the new world or space frontiers. Our unborn, uncharted being awaits to prepare us for our next level of emergence in the life of spirit.

Our period cycles are like tides going in and out, like alternating currents of fullness and emptiness encompassing both the receptivity of fertilization and the bleeding of release. When we complete menopause we move beyond this alternating cyclic nature and become like a direct current, charged and focused with the ability to speak and act truth, and to experience directly who we are through our inner vision. Margaret Mead said that the highest creative force in the universe is the post–menopausal woman. Certainly there is a tremendous shift of energy which is both liberating and powerful. We need to cooperate fully with this process to make the most of this creative opportunity. As attention shifts to the inner world, away from the personal into the universal, we learn to enjoy what is being given in our elder years, and we do not waste time in fear and negativity by longing for what has already passed away.

Spirituality radiates strongly from both the very young and the very old. The love that flows naturally between children and the elderly reflects the world of spirit that we all emerged from at birth and to which we all return at death. Infants and children radiate the softness and innocence of being as yet untouched by life. The elders radiate the wisdom of the life experience and all they have endured, survived and transformed. There is a magic connection between the elders and the young which is enjoyed by both. This loving connection inspires the natural and affectionate sharing of cultural and spiritual values from generation to generation.

There is no more perfect use of this mid–life time than to practice the spiritual life through regular meditation and prayer. Many elderly people complain that they don't sleep as much and don't have as much to do. Make good use this time for devotion. We do not need to mourn that the time for worldly activities is over. We can use this time to build our connection with the divine. We can seek out teachers and develop our inner lives. This will create a magnet of peace, contentment, joy and purpose within that will become a fountainhead to nourish others. We must not miss this opportunity. We can be an example for the young – a guide, explorer, role model, and a graceful, beautiful, wise woman. We can turn our inner face toward God and the divine, and our outer face to the world. Perhaps we can also experience them as one.

Movements of the soul represents a deeper current of truth than flows underneath the obvious, superficial events of our daily lives. We have to see deeper. We have to participate consciously in the journey of our soul as it moves through its soujourn in our bodies. The physical growth and decline of our bodies represents the temporal. Connect with the deeper truth of existence. Dance the flower that is your soul.

# Medical Realities

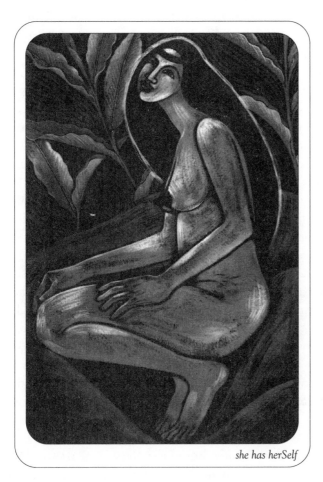

*she has herSelf*

Facing the dragons of modern medicine requires women to have tremedous instincts, the ability to say no, the self–esteem to set limits and ask for what we want and need, and the courage to seek and find humane and appropriate guidance and support for health needs. Now that we have expanded our vision by exploring the many different approaches and perceptions of mid–life, we can return to modern medicine with a fresh perspective and a deeper ground of confidence and responsibility. Disease has many roots, from heredity, past lives, constitutional weaknesses, aging factors, lifestyle and spiritual, mental and emotional causes. While there are disease conditions that we do not seem to be directly responsible for, at least in this life, we have definitely played a part of the creation of most diseases we experience in our elder years. Just as we have contributed to their manifestation, we contribute to their dissolution. Now instead of expecting doctors to make everything come out all right after we have created severe and often life–threatening conditions, we can learn how to prevent diseases. We can also take the time and energy to correct health problems long before they reach the chronic stage. We can appreciate modern medical technical skills and give thanks that they are available should we ever need them. At the same time we can become directly and therapeutically involved in clearing our spiritual, mental and emotional roots of disease. We need to take a higher level responsibility for our own lives and bodies. We can also learn how to adjust our daily lives so that our habits do not create disease.

As modern medicine developed it must have seemed like light emerging out of darkness to the people of the early part of this century. Devoted doctors and scientists discovered germs and created medicines and operations that dramatically saved lives. However, no model is perfect or complete. Because modern medicine developed out of mechanistic and scientific hierarchical thought that did not consider the effect of mind, emotion or spirit on a physical condition, the system itself disregards the whole person and focuses on the physical. Modern medicine also regards the body as a machine and believes that when a part of a machine fails, the efficient treatment is to fix the part or replace it. True healing and the release of deep causes within the life of a person are not addressed. Neither is responsibility is accepted for the effects of radical surgeries and drug therapies on individuals who are left on their own to adjust and recover.

While modern medicine has produced great light in this world it also has a shadow. As a system matures both participants and observers become more aware of what is lacking. Creative researchers seek and find ways to balance and offer what was not included in the system itself. Thus we find the constantly strengthening and growing force of alternative and complementary medicine providing what our medical system does not. Ideally the two systems should work hand in hand to provide the best possible care for the patient. However, there are vested interests that have much to lose if practitioners and doctors are able to prevent illness and therefore reduce the need for medical, hospital and surgical care, or lifetime supplies of medicinal drugs. Instead of medicine being purely a humanitarian service it has become a political machine which invests millions in preserving its monopoly and its power. While we would not like to exist in a world which did not have modern medicine as one of its resources, we also would not like to exist in a world which did not teach correct living habits, educate about the cause and cure of disease, offer therapies that balance and harmonize body energies and functions and help prevent the development of chronic disease. Perhaps the way forward is to combine the best of both systems based on respect for the inherent values of each system, and give the citizens of this democratic society free choice to select a combination of preventive, therapeutic and emergency care.

Orthodox medicine, based as it is on masculine scientific thought, does not respect anything that cannot be seen, measured and proven. Much of life and death is invisible and immeasurable, as are feelings, thoughts and spiritual realities. The definable, measurable realities are only a small part of our life experience. As science approaches these subtler realities, new systems have to be created to embrace them. Future systems of integrated medicine will benefit greatly from these changes in scientific thought.

I believe that modern medicine is fundamentally benevolent, but in my practice I have cared for rejects and failures of the system. I have witnessed many unnecessary sufferings and gross insensitivities on the part of mainstream medical practitioners. I have also worked with wonderful and brilliant doctors who had a great respect for and worked with alternative and complementary practitioners. Over the years I have even welcomed several medical doctors to my study programs in the School of Natural Medicine. As we develop holistic minds and evolve as human beings we will be able to work with and respect others who have different ideas and training. None of us can offer everything and no model is perfect. It is more important to give the best service possible to whatever patient or client comes our way than to believe that only we are right, or that only we have a monopoly on what is possible in the realms of healing, and life and death. We are all servants before the divine forces of this universe, and the more we are able to surrender our limited mental concepts, the better.

Modern medicine is also vulnerable to the dark side of capitalism in the form of factual distortions for the sake of profit. Doctors are constantly exposed to seductive advertising literature from technical and drug companies whose financial existence is dependent upon convincing doctors to use their products. It would be unrealistic to expect medical doctors to be immune to such powerful and sophisticated influences. Furthermore, the doctor must rely on the integrity of multi–national and corporate drug companies to provide medicines that they can use in their practices. Unfortunately there have been more than a few violations of this trust on the part of profit seeking institutions. Human beings have been used as laboratory experiments, often with disastrous results. Also short–term intake of certain drugs may not seem to produce side effects, but we do not have any real way of assessing long–term reactions.

When problems occur with medical products such as the Dalkon Shield or breast implants women suffer, but gynecologists minimize the problems and protect the manufacturers. An excuse that is used is that women must not be frightened unnecessarily. This attitude is mimicked by the press. Lawsuits are settled secretly and the products often continue to be used. The reality is that in many instances the medical profession is riddled with greed and dishonesty. Researchers, manufacturers, regulators and doctors protect each other, rather than their patients.

We are raised to respect doctors and surgeons for their devoted years of study, their sacrifices and their remarkable skills. While this respect should not be eroded, neither should we regard them as having absolute control over our bodies and our lives so that we cannot question or refuse their suggestions for treatment. We need to be fully informed and responsible for the decisions we make, the medicines we accept, or whatever we allow to be done to us. We do not have to surrender ourselves as a victim of modern medicine. We can cooperate fully and intelligently with the best of what is offered medically and also choose to explore educational, therapeutic, natural, alternative and complementary healing.

When women enter mid–life, experience health problems and visit their doctor, the physical aspect of the menopause is magnified to such a degree that the full process of the spiritual unfolding and mental and emotional transformation that is taking place is ignored or disregarded. Causes in life habits are mostly disregarded. Everything is blamed on hormones and the menopause. The ovary is regarded as a failure. The womb becomes redundant. Aging and death are seen as proceeding at rapidly increasing rates without any possibility of regeneration or healing. Unnecessary surgeries and radical treatments are administered without even trying safer and more natural means. Women are having their breasts, ovaries and wombs removed as though this is normal. Synthetic hormones and drugs rule our bodies and women become increasingly distraught and dysfunctional as they lose control over their bodies and their lives.

There is no cultural vision of the wise woman who has successfully weathered the challenges of life to emerge enriched and fulfilled, in charge of her physical, emotional, mental and spiritual being. We have few examples to inspire us with their wisdom. We have to develop our wise woman within to see us through this passage and rely on our inner instinct and strength.

When the change of life is experienced over the background of a severe chronic disease, the picture becomes confused. Menopause is often blamed for lifestyle, aging and disease symptoms. The concern for survival and the fulfillment of day–to–day responsibilities has often been so all–consuming that women may not have taken the time to take care of their health or even to understand what health means. Because mid–life is a time of harvest, problems surface demanding resolution. Somehow we must find the time and energy to give to ourselves as we move through this passage. We must nurture and support this life passage that prepares us for our future as an elder. Physically we may be waning but spiritually we have the potential to open like a lover before the divine. However much we have given of ourselves to our loved ones, our husbands, our children, our work and our world, now is the time to give to ourselves.

We must find strength in the face of the challenges that emerge for us, whether they be physical, emotional, mental or spiritual. These challenges can be regarded as dragons that we must fight, and then as partners that we dance with as we surrender to the lesson and attain our victory. There is no right. There is no wrong. There is only love. Whatever we do with whatever we have in front of us is the best we can do. Only that is right. We do not need to compare ourselves to anyone else. Our own life journey is all that matters. There are many realities we can be part of. Mid–life is the time to recognize and live from our own reality.

When we interact with doctors and the medical system we must challenge them to expand and grow. We must also demand communication and respect. We must find the courage to seek and find those who will help us. We must overcome our feelings of fear, helplessness and despair. Whatever is not being provided on the outside we have the inner resources to provide. But we must awaken those visionary strengths within us. It is not always someone or something on the outside that will save us or help us. We must seek and find that help and that grace within our own being.

Menopausal symptoms can be very confusing. Because we are also emotionally and mentally challenged, the physical problems can seem more drastic. We can choose to believe that everything that is happening is raw fuel for our spiritual awakening, and accept each challenge from this perspective. Menopausal symptoms can also become confused with chronic aging and disease conditions that increase their intensity. Irregular cycles of menopausal pain, bleeding and ovulation may be more painful or more uncomfortable. However, if the holistic causes of the disease are recognized, resolved and released, pressures ease within our interior ecology. If we take an interest in our bodies, we can nurture them back to health. If we make a determination we can heal even chronic and supposedly incurable conditions. We can reach out our antennae into the universe and seek and find the love, support and nourishment that we

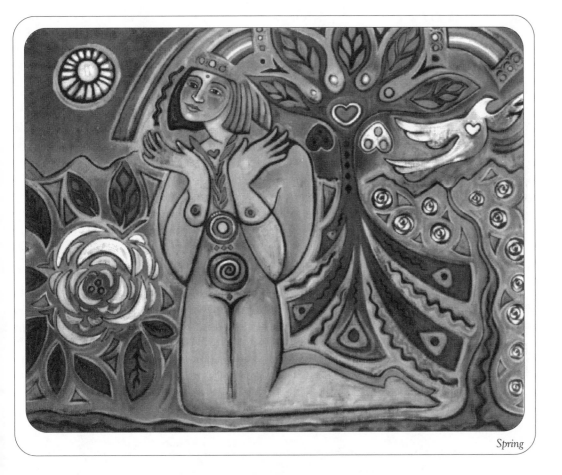

Spring

need. We can continue growing instead of feeling like our lives are over. Like the phoenix, we can rise from the ashes of our growing unfolding center. We can release the past and give birth to ourselves into the next cycle of our lives.

Reproductive operations create shock and infection, inhibit the flow of blood and lymph, affect hormones and bring on aging and menopause earlier than necessary. When an ovary is removed it alters the flow of pelvic blood supply and stresses the remaining ovary. When the uterus is removed the ovaries shut down earlier. Whenever there is a total hysterectomy, there is profound shock to the entire being, as well as instant menopause. Estrogen drugs or natural estrogens from herbs and foods become necessary whenever radical surgery has been performed.

While we must give appreciation to the medical profession for its great skill and for the lives it saves and extends once disease has reached chronic and life-threatening status, we cannot condone or excuse the lack of education, concern and healing that should be given in the early stages. The medical profession resists the legalization of natural medicine and alternative therapeutics and does not consider that it is patients who will benefit from preventive and healing care. There would probably be less need for drugs, hospitalization, surgery, chemotherapy and radiation, and therefore less income for the medical profession and hospitals. Perhaps people who now study to become doctors might become alternative care practitioners if natural medicine was legalized and supported by the citizens of this country, the government, doctors, hospitals and insurance companies. Instead of waiting for conditions to reach disaster level where dramatic and life saving operations are necessary, as well as very expensive, the therapists, professional health educators and doctors would cooperate to support human beings to lead healthy lives. The emphasis would shift to health education and prevention.

It is a natural human trait to be afraid of change because of the fear of loss. Adjustments would take place as our society allowed the integration of prevention and healing into its orthodox system. However, integration of the scientific and the natural, the left and right brain approaches, would help this world to become a better place. Healthy people with harmonious inner lives can make positive contributions to this world. True health can be our right.

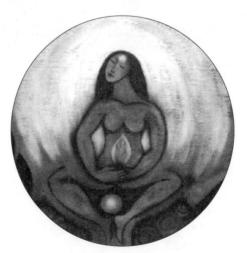

# The Honored Elder

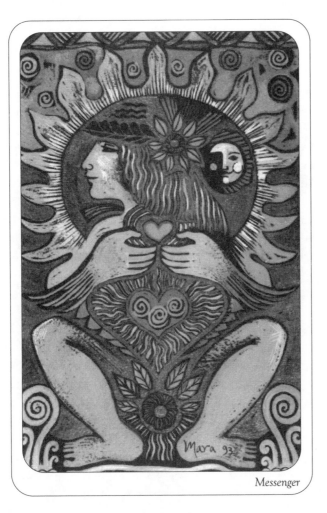

Messenger

If we survive mid–life by cooperating creatively with the process, we emerge fully born. We have become a fully integrated human being, still feminine in our physical body, but beyond traditionally defined gender sexuality. The strength and power of this integration, the lightness attained by the clearing and the release, and the wisdom gained by direct experience with the energies awakened within, give women a foundation that supports spirituality and our highest purpose. We have united the opposites within – youth and old age, masculine and feminine, earth and heaven, knowledge and wisdom – and we are ready to continue the journey of our soul.

Wisdom is now our path. We have learned to accept, adjust and accommodate ourselves to whatever comes before us. We no longer fight or resist our destiny, because we have learned to make the most of every opportunity and life situation. We no longer need to seek love from the world because we exist in a state of love. We have achieved our life purpose and become a true human being.

Because we faced the health challenges during our mid–life, we have learned how to become independently healthy. We have the practical tools, information and support system to deal with any problems that may come up. We have learned to live moderately and simply and have included the realities of healthy preventive living into our lifestyle. We have become masters of our own bodies and our own lives, even though we are still a student of our own lives. We have learned how to live, and we have learned how to die.

There will not even be the question "What will I do with the rest of my life?" There is so much unfolding to experience within and without. Our lives have become our greatest creativity. All around us, and in everything we do, our world benefits from our achievements. The work of integration has been achieved and our path out of this world lies before us. Every day we are closer to our departure from our bodies and our lives. Each day we have the opportunity to live in the present moment with love. Each day we prepare for our departure by awakening our spirituality. The journey of our soul in this world began at birth and it is completed when we return to our source. We live a divine mystery and to a divine mystery we return.

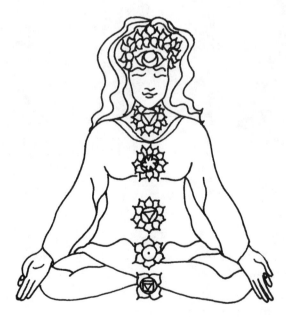

# GLOSSARY

AMENORRHEA: Periodic absence of blood flow during menopause is normal. However, abnormal cessation of menses due to low body fat caused by extreme stress, starvation, intense exercise and eating disorders, requires treatment.

CORPUS LUTEUM: Whenever an egg is released from the wall of the ovary a swelling of yellow, hormone–producing tissue occurs and encourages the production of progesterone.

DYSMENORRHEA: abnormally difficult or painful menstruation.

ESTROGEN: A constellation of over two dozen steroidal hormones, estrogen is produced in different areas of the body such as the ovaries, adrenals, from androstenedione in the body fat cells, and during pregnancy, in the placenta and fetus. Stimulated by pituitary hormones, Luteinizing Hormone (LH) and Follicle Stimulating Hormone (FSH), estrogen triggers ovulation. If Estrogen Replacement Therapy (ERT) is taken it is essential that natural progesterone also be given, otherwise endometrial and vaginal carcinomas can occur. Excess estrogen also blocks the thyroid, increases water retention and helps to cause ovarian fibroid tumors and cysts. It also can create health problems for women who have had a history of liver disorders or malfunction.

FOLLICLE STIMULATING HORMONE: FSH is produced by the pituitary to stimulate ovulation. FSH rises during menopause and remains high after menopause.

LUTEINIZING HORMONE: LH is produced by the pituitary together with FSH to stimulate estrogen production in the ovaries and trigger ovulation, changing the ovum follicle into corpus luteum. LH rises during menopause and remains high after menopause unless excesses of pineal melatonin inhibit production. Melatonin is produced at night only in complete darkness.

MENORRHAGIA: Excess blood flow occurs during menopause because of cysts, fibroids, polyps, IUD problems, hyperplasia (the increase in the number of cells in an area), endometriosis and hormonal imbalances. When progesterone levels stay high during the month, the endometrium continues to grow, filling the uterus with blood and eventually flooding out in gushes and clots. This flooding can continue for many days, causing exhaustion due to loss of blood and anemia.

PROGESTERONE: A constellation of steroidal hormones produced in small amounts by the adrenals, in the corpus luteum after ovulation and by the placenta, progesterone is produced when ovulation occurs. Because ovulation slows down, becomes irregular and eventually ceases during menopause, progesterone levels decrease. This affects bone formation and in some cases helps to create osteoporosis. Natural progesterone, a cholesterol derivative, is found in vegetables, Mexican yams and soybeans. Chemical progestagens confuse female bodies which produce less natural progesterone as a result, and further helps to cause hypoglycemia, fluid retention, salt imbalances and pre–menstrual symptoms. Progesterone helps prevent the undesirable effects of excess estrogen such as uterine and breast cysts and cancer.

This is a guide to herbs which are directly related to hormones, feminine reproductive organs, monthly cycles and menopause. Herbs can be used in different ways: in teas, tinctures, powders, capsules or tablets, as individual herbs or blended in formulae. Because my approach is based on the individual I do not give specific dosage recommendations. I recommend consulting a professional herbalist, buying well known organic products which contain these herbs, studying herbs, and reading herbals such as *Herbs of Grace*, for specific guidance. It is my experience that herbs work best whenthey are blended into combinations which support the inner ecology of the body. Asking an individual hormone herb to work against constipation, lymphatic congestion or liver disorders, for example, is asking too much. Treatment for symptoms is most effective when it includes the cause at the constitutional, eliminative and inner ecology levels.

ALFALFA– *Medicago sativa*: **a hormone balancer; contains phytoestrogens** that act either as estrogen enhancers or balancers; when estrogen is low they stimulate estrogen activity; when there is too much estrogen they occupy the site, reducing estrogen activity.

ANGELICA – *Angelica acutiloba* and *archangelica*: **relaxes smooth muscles including uterine antispasmodic action**, and bronchial and intestinal spasmolytic effects; also anti-allergic, enhances immune action, is anti-tumor and antibacterial; *Angelica archangelica* can be a substitute for Dong Quai, as well as offering digestive and respiratory benefits, although because the roots are only two years old they are not as strong in their hormonal effect as Panax Ginseng or Dong Quai.

BLACK COHOSH – *Cimicifuga racemosa*: an anti-inflammatory herb which **promotes estrogenic hormonal actions**; traditionally used in gynecology, it relieves dysmenorrhea; good for patients when rheumatism or nerve, bone, joint and muscle pain accompany gynecological or menopausal symptoms; also an excellent homeopathic female remedy.

BLACK HAW BARK – *Viburnum prunifolium*: specific for the female reproductive organs; can be used interchangeably with Cramp Bark; **relieves uterine cramping;** antispasmodic; hypotensive; relieves dysmenorrhea; specific in threatened miscarriage; relieves spasms in the fallopian tubes, thus facilitating conception during hypertonicity.

CHASTEBERRY – *Vitex agnus castus*: **increases leutinizing hormone (LH)**; inhibits release of follicle stimulating hormone (FSH), thus **promoting progesterone** and the corpus luteum; increases fertility; balances irregular cycles; relieves premenstrual fluid retention; improves acne.

CRAMP BARK – *Viburnum opulus*: general female reproductive antispasmodic useful during **painful cramps** and when miscarriage is a possibility.

DONG QUAI – *Angelica sinensis*: **restores female reproductive balance**; increases fertility; **estrogenic** properties benefits the follicular phase of the monthly flow; increases blood loss, so do not use when there is already excessive bleeding; use when bleeding is over, both as a tonic and to replace what has been lost through menstrual blood; can be both an abortifacient, or a relaxant; use as a tonic during the first three months of pregnancy; relaxes muscles; hypotensive to bronchials, intestines and to uterus; anti-allergic; anti-bacterial; anti-tumor; enhances immunity.

FALSE UNICORN ROOT – *Chamaelirium luteum* or previously *Helonias dioica*: reproductive tonic and strengthener; contains **estrogenic steroidal saponins**; balances irregular cycles; stops threatened abortion; use for reproductive or hormonal treatment when there are digestive or liver problems.

HOPS – *Humulus lupulus*: mild sedative which relieves insomnia; **active estrogenic**; a digestive bitter tonic which improves digestion, assimilation and abdominal circulation, resulting in balanced menstruation; specific for the estrogenic follicular phase; mild anodyne and sedative properties relieve dysmenorrhea; aids the constitution while relieving symptoms.

LADY'S MANTLE – *Alchemilla vulgaris*: **progesteronic** female reproductive herb; best given ten to fifteen days before menstruation; increases circulation to the reproductive organs; balances hormones; astringent; antihemorrhagic.

LICORICE ROOT – *Glycyrrhiza glabra*: **phytoestrogen**, amphoteric balancer when menstrual cycles are irregular; **inhibits high estrogen and activates deficient estrogen**; induces normal ovulation; fluid retention rarely occurs when used only in the first half of the monthly cycle; in severe fluid retention cases it can be left out; anti-inflammatory; increases immunity and liver activity.

MOTHERWORT– *Leonurus cardiaca*: **relieves uterine pain** or atony especially when aggravated by nervous tension, emotional trauma, stress and anxiety; antispasmodic; hypotensive, sedative; amphoteric balance; slightly stimulating to uterus and intestines; relaxing **emmenagogue** that reduces afterpains; a galactagogue that stimulates breast milk flow.

POMEGRANATE SEEDS – *Punica granatum*: ancient fertility symbol associated with the myth of Persephone; **contains estrone** which is identical with the estrogen hormone.

PULSATILLA – *Anemone pulsatilla*: often used homeopathically, it has **progesterone properties**; specific pelvic anodyne; both stimulating and relaxing to pelvic organs; used in constitutional formulae, but also separately for quick pain relief; give when depression and irritability are related to nervous tension in the female reproductive organs; for weepy women with wandering mind and depleted nervous system; low dosage is effective; relieves dysmenorrhea, ovarian pain, and endometriosis; **caution**: take with food to avoid gastrointestinal irritation.

SAGE – *Salvia officinalis* (not the Artemesias or Sagebrush varieties): decreases secretions of mother's milk, sweat and therefore **hot flashes; contains estrogenic substances**; useful as an antiaphrodesiac and to reduce excess or leaking sperm flow; antioxidant useful as an aging preventative; carminative, antispasmodic; stimulates digestive fluids; volatile oil is antimicrobial; high in zinc.

SAINT JOHN'S or JOAN'S WORT – *Hypericum perforatum*: antidepressive when used over two to three months, lightens moods, even producing euphoria; **excellent for chronic pelvic conditions with an emotional or mental tension and nervous cause**; useful for chronic urinary infections and whenever there is suppression of urine; relieves delayed menses or menopausal neurosis; antiviral; tumor inhibitors; it is being used successfully in HIV positive and AIDS cases; a widely used homeopathic remedy.

SARSAPARILLA – *Smilax ornata* and *officinalis*: **contains hormonal precursors for progesterone;** a rheumatic and skin alterative; binds endotoxins in the intestines, reducing metabolic stress on the eliminative organs; useful in dysentery, syphilis and mercury poisoning.

SIBERIAN GINSENG – *Eleuthrococcus senticosus*: adaptogenic, nonspecific immune enhancing; **regulates hormone release**; relieves cellular level stress; prevents viral illness and improves health performance during stress from climate, pathology and physical demands; positively affects the hypothalamus discriminating center in the brain.

SQUAW VINE – *Mitchella repens*: a greatly respected Native American herb; specific for pregnancy preparation, maintenance and birthing; **regulates uterine and ovarian dysfunction**; increases circulation; relieves congestion and irritation in the reproductive organs; relaxes the nervous system; diuretic; used topically to relieve the sore nipples of nursing mothers.

WILD YAM ROOT – *Dioscorea*: **contains progesterone precursors** (diosgenin and pregnenolone); forms the basis of contraceptives and steroidal hormones made by drug companies; anti-inflammatory because of hormonal precursors to cortisone; spasmolytic; relieves afterpains, dysmenorrhea, and ovarian neuralgia.

YARROW – *Achillea millefolium*: anti-inflammatory, carminative, choleretic, digestive stimulant, spasmolytic; contains thujone, a uterine stimulant; active homeostatic agent; an **ideal female reproductive balancer** for menstrual regulation and to stimulate or relax the uterus in deficient or excess flow; assists digestive and liver function to metabolize estrogens; reduces inflammation; relieves uterine spasms; effective when treating chronic conditions.

## SUPPLEMENT INFORMATION

It is essential to read every supplement and herb information label carefully and thoroughly and ask the staff of stores where supplements and bottled herbs are purchased to recommend those labels that are made from organic living food grown material. Recommended labels for this quality and integrity are Rainbow Light Living Source, New Chapter and Megafood. Minerals are often better absorbed when they are taken in their homeopathic or biochemic tissue salt form. Alternatively, look in the *Herbs of Grace* book and order fresh herb powders that are high sources for the vitamins and mineral necessary for your healing. The retail order form is included in the appendices.

# MENOPAUSAL SUPPORTIVE HERBS

*'Make these herbs your menopausal companions.'*

These herbs blend well into teas. Milk Thistle can be taken as directed.

BORAGE – *Borago officinalis succus:* hormonally active, it **supports the functions of estrogenic and progesteronic herbs because of its adrenal and nutritive functions**; excellent to take after steroid treatments, which weaken the adrenals; an ancient courage remedy, it dispels melancholy and gladdens the heart; Borage seeds are the **highest source of linolenic acid;** anti-inflammatory; high levels of calcium and potassium support the heart; galactagogue (breast milk stimulant); fresh Borage juice is an excellent way to receive the benefits of this herb; the flowers are beautiful in salads, but remove the rough parts first.

DANDELION – *Taraxacum officinalis radix:* use the root for hepatobiliary choleretic and **liver restorative** functions; nutritive; assists the liver in cleansing and hormone metabolizing functions; for best results alternate with Oregon Grape root; use the leaves as a diuretic and to avoid potassium depletion; contains 4.25% potassium; balances premenstrual cycle.

HORSETAIL – *Equisetum arvense:* rich in silica, it supports bone growth; reverses osteoporosis; heals gum disease; rich in flavinoids, it eases hot flashes; increases circulation; reduces bloating; relieves; relaxes at the same time as it increases energy.

MILK THISTLE – *Silybum marianum semen:* **detoxifies and protects the liver;** take as powder, one tablespoon daily, for three weeks of the month, except when bleeding.

NETTLES – *Urtica dioica, Urtica urens:* the ideal menopause friend; **supports bones;** stabilizes blood sugar; reduces fatigue and headaches; **nourishes and strengthens the kidneys and adrenals;** improves skin and hair - and this is not all that it does!

OATSTRAW – *Avena sativa:* another menopause friend that works wonders in many different areas such as energy, heart, bones, teeth, blood sugar, nervous system, sleep, bladder difficulties and circulation; caution – don't take this herb if there is extreme exhaustion.

OREGON GRAPE ROOT – *Berberis aquifolium:* stimulates the liver and bile; aids the liver in hormone metabolism and elimination; leave it out of progesterone formulae because it might prevent disruption of ovum implantation since it also stimulates the uterus.

VALERIAN – *Valeriana sitchensis* or *officinalis:* **relieves anxiety,** pain and physical, emotional and mental stress; antispasmodic; hypotensive, anti-inflammatory, somewhat anesthetic; useful for endometriosis.

VERVAIN – *Verbena offinalis:* **relieves depression, tension and stress** related muscle and uterine tension; good for the premenstrual phase especially when combined with a hepatic stimulant.

# HORMONAL HERBS FOR MENOPAUSE

### Hormone Balancing Herbs

Alfalfa, Black Cohosh, Chasteberry, Cramp bark, Dandelion, Dong Quai, False Unicorn Fenugreek, Hops, Licorice, Liferoot, Motherwort, Nettles, Raspberry leaves, Red Clover blossoms Sage, Sarsaparilla, Saw Palmetto, Wild Yam root, Yarrow.

### Estrogen Producing Herbs – *when menses are early, irregular or scanty*

Alfalfa, Black Cohosh root, Dong Quai, False Unicorn Root, Hops, Licorice, Sage, Sweet Briar hips or leaf buds, Pomegranate seeds, Red Clover flowers and leaves, herbs containing flavinoid (the inner skin of citrus fruits), Buckwheat greens and sprouts, Yellow Dock leaves, Elder berries and flowers, Hawthorn, Horsetail, Knotweeds, Roses, Shepherd's Purse, Sea Buckthorn, Toadflax and White Dead Nettle.

### Progesterone Promoting Herbs – *when menses come too frequently*

Alfalfa, Chasteberry, Lady's Mantle, Pulsatilla, Sarsaparilla, Wild Yam root, Yarrow.

** Caution – Leave Oregon Grape root out of any progesterone formulas.

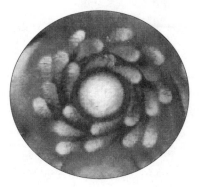

# MENOPAUSAL SUPPORTIVE SUPPLEMENTS & FOODS

ANTIOXIDANTS: natural substances that prevent oxygen deterioration such as amino acids, vitamins A, B1, B2, C and E, beta carotene, inositol, lecithin, selenium and zinc, help support healthy liver and kidney function, so necessary for vitamin D metabolism.

BEE POLLEN: a potent food which offers superior nutrition, it is a complete protein which contains all twenty-two amino acids; it is rich in A, B, C and E vitamins, as well as offering high levels of coenzymes, enzymes and other minerals; sprinkle it on all your foods or blend into drinks.

CALCIUM: a necessary ingredient for all cycles of a woman's life, calcium is especially important during menopause to prevent bone problems and osteoporosis, as well as to help prevent hot flashes, gum and tooth disease and nervous disorders; use herbs and food sources that include the other minerals and vitamins necessary for complete digestion and assimilation, such as Comfrey, Hawthorn berries, Licorice, Horsetail, Marshmallow and Red Clover blossoms, as well as almonds, seaweeds, sesame seeds, soybeans, kale and turnips.

EVENING PRIMROSE OIL: a high source of gamma-linolenic acid (GLA), one of the fatty acids needed by the body to make prostaglandins, which are found in every cell of the body and are involved in many diverse functions to do with circulation, reproduction, metabolism and growth; all prostaglandins are synthesized instantaneously from two essential fatty acids (EFA's): linoleic acid and alpha linolenic acids; Black Currant and Borage oils are also high sources of GLA.

*Iron*: a metabolic energizer, iron is found in every cell of the body; when iron is deficient the cells cannot get enough oxygen, blood quality suffers, and exhaustion results; take the Anemia formula and make sure you eat enough high iron foods such as dulse seaweed, wheat and rice bran, wheat germ, sesame seeds, pumpkin and squash.

MANGANESE: a component of female sex hormones, manganese helps prevent osteoporosis; high sources are Comfrey, Cramp bark, Gravel root, Oat straw, and Uva Ursi herbs, as well as apples, peaches, turnips and rye.

SEAWEEDS: provide alkaline nutrition high in concentrated trace minerals, calcium and vitamins, which are particularly effective for nourishing and balancing the endocrine glands.

SPIRULINA: a blue-green algae of harmonious microorganisms which provides superior nutrients high in usable protein, B vitamins and gamma–linolenic acid (GLA); reduces hunger.

VITAMIN B 6: eases PMS anxiety and reduces water retention; essential for women using oral contraceptives because it reduces the phlebitis risk; high sources are spirulina and sprouts.

VITAMIN D: in its active hormonal form, vitamin D improves and protects bone density; we can receive vitamin D from sunbathing, Alfalfa and Fenugreek herbs and apple and watercress.

VITAMIN E: a nutrient that oxygenates body cells, it is also a female reproductive remedy which relieves cramping, hot flashes and vaginal dryness; high natural sources are Alfalfa, Flax seeds, Marigold, Peppermint, Rose hips, wheat germ oil, parsley, and watercress.

# DIETARY SUPPORT FOR MENOPAUSE

## AVOID

Alcohol
Animal products
Caffeine
Chocolate
Dairy products
Environmental pollution
Fast foods
Fats (some is necessary)
Fried foods and unsaturated oils
Foods that create reactions and allergies
Medications like aspirin, sleeping pills, tranqullizers, pain pills
Proteins in excess, whether meat, beans or tofu
Salt
Simple carbohydrates
Spicy foods
Sugar
Recreational drugs
Tobacco
White flour products

## REMEMBER

Alcohol decreases liver capabilities, suppresses bone growth, upsets ovarian
   function and increases the likelihood of menstrual irregularities
Excessive protein diets increase the secretion of calcium through the urine
Excessive salt increases the secretion of calcium through the urine
Caffeine increases calcium loss and neutralizes the metabolism of iron
Junk foods and caffeine also leach calcium from the bones.

## INCREASE

Simplicity
Freshness
Fresh local organic fruits
Fresh organic juices
Nuts
Seeds
Fresh local organic vegetables
Whole grains

# MENOPAUSE SYMPTOMS & CONDITIONS

Information and natural treatment suggestions on these symptoms and conditions can be found in the Physical Healing – Symptoms section in alphabetical order on the above pages.

# HERBAL FORMULAS & TREATMENTS

## CREATE A RELATIONSHIP WITH YOUR HERBS

Before taking your herbs create a relationship with them and welcome them into your life. Put them in a special container and visualize their healing energy. It is important to regard them as nourishment, so that you can receive them, digest them, and assimilate thems. Make them a part of your life – read herb books, grow them in gardens and look for them in the countryside. Plants are our friends and helpers. They lead us toward health and healing.

As you measure the herbs, capsule them, make them into pills and take them with your meals, treat them with love and respect. The quality of your energy will mix with the herbs. Look with eyes of love, and receive their contribution to your life with gratitude.

The herbal formulas given in this book are nutritional, non–toxic, non–habit–forming herbal nutrients. They are gentle and balancing. Pay attention and monitor your body's changes. Ask your practitioner for help if you are not sure about something. Education, guidance, and communication are an essential part of any treatment.

## HERBAL POWDERS

In our Herbs of Grace pharmacy and dispensary we prepare the herbal formulas in powder form from wildcrafted organic herbs in small amounts so that they are fresh. Because we believe they are more effective and potent in their pure state, we do not tincture them or send them to factories to be bound with fillers, to be heated or pressure tableted. We provide fresh, pure, unprocessed herbs from plants growing in their natural habitat.

We encourage you to involve yourself in the preparation of your herbs. You are welcome to prepare the formulas for your own use by following the proportions given in this book. We believe that if you become involved in your own healing by making your own herbal tablets or capsules, you are increasing the positive healing energy of the herbs. It is important to recognize that time, love and energy focused on the herbs increases their ability to contribute to your health and well–being.

If you cannot take powders in liquid or in capsules because of difficulty swallowing or because of a sensitive digestive system, you can swallow them with a Slippery Elm drink, mix the dry herbs with honey, melted butter or Slippery Elm, or make tinctures or extracts from the powders. You receive greater value for money with fresh herbs because you are not paying for expensive manufacturing processes, packaging, advertising, storage, shipping and sales commissions.

If you are going to make up your own formula, buy fresh, wildcrafted organic herbs and grind them in an electric coffee mill or a Vita Mix. Some herbs are so hard that you will not be able to grind them and you may have to pulverize them in some other way, or purchase them in powdered form. It takes effort and investment to set up your own herbal pharmacy and to research sources for all the herbs required in the formula.

# Information & Cautions

*Practitioner Information*

Because several formulas are combined into personal nutrient mixes, using from five to nine formulas mixed together to balance the inner ecology, stimulating hot herbs have been deleted from many of the formulas. If a formula is used individually and does not contain stimulating herbs such as Cayenne, Garlic or Ginger, these may be added whenever they are needed.

*Allergy Cautions*

If you are sensitivite to hot sprices or have liver reactions to fried foods, oils or fats make up the formula without any of the strong hot herbs such as Cayenne, Ginger, Cloves, Garlic, and Ginseng. You can also test yourself or your client with a pendulum or kineseology.

*Digestive Cautions*

If there is digestive sensitivity it is wise to take the herbs with a warm drink made from one teaspoon of Slippery Elm mixed with one cup of warm water, or soy, rice or almond milk, and honey. This soothes their passage through the stomach and intestines until the healing of the gastrointestinal tract has strengthened the system.

*When To Take the Herbs*

Take the herbs immediately before eating so that the saliva and digestive juices mix the herbs with the food. If you forget and take them after your meal, eat more food right after taking the herbs. If you do not have a full meal three times a day, take the herbs with a healthy snack. You can also take them more often. As long as the daily dose of herbs is taken throughout the day, suit yourself as to how often or when. Do not take them on an empty stomach until your system is used to them. Eventually most people can take them with water or juice, or even when on a fast. Best results are achieved when herbs are combined with restorative changes in diet and living habits.

Manufacturers make them in various sizes. We recommend capsule size '0' or '00'. Capsules are readily available in drugstore pharmacies and health food stores in non–vegetarian gelatin form. It is also possible to purchase capsules made of a vegetable or seaweed gel in most health food stores. There are two ways of filling capsules which are described below.

*Herbal Brews*

The Chinese method of brewing herbs may also be used if warm herbal tea is preferred. Put the daily dose in a container and pour boiling water over it, then mix and steep. Drink throughout the day. The continuous influence of the tastes on the tongue is beneficial

Experiment and try different methods. Be flexible. At different times it may be preferable to take the powders in different ways.

## CAPSULING

Capsules are small cylindrical containers into which the powdered herb is compressed. We recommend capsule size 'O' or 'OO' Capsules are readily available in drugstore pharmacies and health food stores in non-vegetarian gelatin or vegetable or seaweed gel. There are two ways of filling capsules which are described below.

### Capsuling Method 1:

Put the powders in a dish at least one half to one inch deep. Open the capsule, holding one half in each hand. Press each half of the capsule down into the powder, and tap several times so that the powder is pressed up inside. When both parts of the capsule are as full as possible press the two halves together again to make a finished edible capsule. Do not scoop as this will make the powder fly like dust.

### Capsuling Method 2:

Purchase a capsuling device from a health food store or the Herbs of Grace pharmacy.

## OTHER METHODS OF POWDER PREPARATION

*Honey Tablets*

Make up the honey pills in daily amounts, because there are no preservatives. Pinch off the dose and roll between the fingers before swallowing. Take the pills immediately before eating.

*Butter Tablets*

This ancient Indian method of pill making is easy and pleasant. Mix the powder in melted ghee or butter, shape into a roll and refrigerate. Cut and roll into smooth round pillules.

*Slippery Elm Tablets*

Mix one day's dose of powder with approximately one–third Slippery Elm, add distilled water, form into a roll of herbal compound and then pinch off into pills to roll between your fingers. Make only enough for each day because there is no preservative in the mixture.

*Drinking Powders*

Some people prefer to take the powders straight, either with juice, water, liquid yogurt or soy milk. Mix the powder in just enough liquid to blend, swallow quickly and follow with a chaser. Others report that a straw works wonders well.

The bitter taste contributes healing benefits because it influences the taste buds on the tongue, causing reflex stimulation to the gastrointestinal tract. Because we have unbalanced tastes due to excessive cravings for sweet, salt or sour, the bitter and pungent tastes help balance the taste buds and our digestive processes. According to Ayurveda philosophy it is essential for good health to have all five tastes available regularly in our diet. After a week this method becomes easier. We recommend it whenever possible, except when capsules or tablets are more convenient for work or travel.

# DOSAGE

*Average Monthly Dose*

An average dose for an adult of medium size with reasonable health is about one to two ounces of herbs per week. This makes the monthly dose anywhere from four to eight ounces. This can be increased if the person is large or very active or wishes to pursue a dedicated program of purification and regeneration. The amount can also be increased if higher amounts of nutritional or rejuvenative herbs, such as the Multi–Mineral Vitamins Naturally, Stomach Acid Alkaline, Adrenal or Nerve formula are required. Several different formula are mixed together to provide nutrients to balance the inner ecology. Start off with an average amount and then adjust according to response.

*Chronic Monthly Dose*

Doses for chronic conditions such as arthritis, rheumatism, colitis or nervous exhaustion can be as high as three ounces per week. The exact doseage depends on digestive capability, food habits, symptoms, age, pain levels and other considerations which should be evaluated by a skilled practitioner.

*How to Work Out the Daily Dose*

1. Mix the combination of herbs and formulas appropriate for your constitution, condition, age and size.
2. Divide the herbal powders equally into four plastic baggies, one bag for each week of the month.
3. Take one week's bag and divide the powders into seven piles, one for each day.
4. Once you have worked out the daily dose, divide it by two, three or more, depending on how many times you wish to take the herbs with food during the day.
5. Decide how you wish to take the herbs, then prepare them in daily or weekly amounts.
6. Take individual doses immediately before meals, or with the first bite or two of food.
7. Do not swallow the herbs more than two minutes before eating, or at the end of the meal. If you forget and take them after a meal, eat more food after swallowing the herbs.
8. Once you know your daily amount for this series of herbs there is no need to divide any more of the weekly bags. Take the daily dose with food two or more times a day.

# HERBAL FORMULAS

These herbal formulas are balancing, nutritional, non–toxic and non–habit–forming. They are a highly superior and specific form of natural nutrition to be taken either during a course of purification and rejuvenation or as nutritional supplements.

Individual organs, body systems and glands are restored to normal function when supportive blends of activating, eliminating and rejuvenating herbs are provided. The body takes what it needs, when and where it needs it, from the nutrients offered in the herbal formulas.

Please take the herbs under the guidance of a Natural Physician, Naturopath or Herbalist.

*Formula Proportions*

All herbs are combined in equal parts except where otherwise stated in parentheses, i.e. (0.5) means half a part. The sample formula below means: 6 parts Horsetail, 4 parts Oatstraw, 3 parts Comfrey, 1 part Lobelia, 2 parts Marshmallow root, 1 part Kelp, 1 part Parsley root.

*Horsetail (6), Oatstraw (4), Comfrey (3), Lobelia, Marshmallow root (2), Kelp
and Parsley root*

## ADRENAL FORMULA

Whenever there is continual stress, nervous tension, anxiety and hyperactivity, the adrenal glands become exhausted. This formula provides the nutrients to strengthen, support and rebuild the adrenal glands whenever you are in conflict, face deadlines, emergencies, trauma, or long–term survival flight–or–fight stress.

Adrenal and nerve herbs will help you to become aware of depletion and exhaustion, especially if the use of stimulants are discontinued. It is important to rest and avoid unnecessary activities. Do not push the river; learn to flow with it.

*Borage, Mullein, Lobelia, Ginseng, Gotu Kola, Hawthorn berries and Parsley root*

## ALKALINE FORMULA

"From the ocean cometh all life," Dr. Shook says in his *Treatise on Herbology*, inspiring respect for the nutritional value of seaweeds, which contain almost the full range of basic nutrients that are required by the human body. The body selects what it needs. A valuable source of trace elements, this formula is effective whenever there is an imbalance of chemistry, or a lack of some essential mineral or trace element. This formula will help to balance acid/alkaline, normalize body chemistry, relieve arthritis and rheumatism, and improve nutritional imbalances. It is also useful as an additive in herbal tablet making or poultices because its hygroscopic properties help to form a cohesive mixture.

*Irish Moss, Kelp, Iceland Moss and Bladderwrack*

## ALLERGY FORMULA

Whenever the immune system is overburdened the body reacts to aggravating stimuli with acute reactions such as hay fever, rashes or uncomfortable mucus discharges. Although it is essential to adjust diet and living habits, the force of the discomfort can be alleviated with this formula. There is no substitute for treating the cause of the distress, so unless the body system is cleared and returned to balanced function a true cure cannot take place. For best results use this formula for foundation level treatment in combination with other formulas for restoration of active normal function of the eliminative channels and regeneration of any weak or unbalanced body glands, systems and organs.

*Black Pepper, Burdock root, Cinnamon, Elecampagne, Ephaedra, Ginger root, Licorice root and Marshmallow root*

## ANEMIA FORMULA

This formula provides strength and power to a sluggish system and helps to restore an adequate supply of iron necessary for body metabolism and energy. Especially valuable to pregnant and nursing mothers, this formula provides assimilable iron that does not cause side effects such as constipation. The formula contains all the additional ingredients to utilize the iron in the system. Avoid caffeine in any form when you are iron deficient because it leaches iron from your body. Also avoid it when you are taking iron herbs because it neutralizes the buildup of increased iron.

*Barberry, Comfrey root, Sarsaparilla, Sassafras, Cayenne, Quassia root, Yellow Dock root and Lobelia (0.5)*

## ANTIBIOTICS NATURALLY FORMULA

Whenever acute distress requires strong activation of the lymphatic immune defense system, this formula provides an alternative to synthetic antibiotics, if used in combination with naturopathic first aid techniques and an understanding of the body cleansing required to relieve obstructions to faulty elimination. It is essential that the bowels are cleansed with enemas and stomach juices are neutralized and purified with Peppermint and Thyme tea. Hot Mustard baths that are followed by steaming under quilts will produce a copious skin elimination which will relieve a burdened system. Other complementary treatments are recommended depending on whether there is fever, sore throat, pain, cough, nausea, inflammation or swelling. It is also important to consult your practitioner.

This formula cannot work effectively when there are toxic accumulations, but if the elimination is activated, and the patient is cleansing with herb teas, lemon water and/or fresh juice, there is an excellent chance of overcoming symptoms in a natural way.

Tablet, capsule and tincture dosage can be increased in both amount and frequency during an acute crisis. When dental surgery pierced through the root of my tooth and caused a severe infection, I took doses of twenty–four capsules every half hour, about one hundred fifty capsules per day, for a period of four days. My dentist was amazed when the infection was completely cleared up without an abscess. I received the additional benefit of a complete inner–cleanse, so instead of being depleted by an acute illness, I was rejuvenated and restored. These are the benefits of living with nature's natural pharmacy. Every health problem becomes a learning challenge which leaves one with greater understanding to apply in any future situation.

This formula can effectively be combined with my Sore Throat Syrup: simmer hot water, honey, apple cider vinegar, lemon juice, Garlic, Ginger and Cayenne pepper. Gargle thoroughly and then drink. Adjust the proportions according to taste preferences. This combination neutralizes the strong flavors, resulting in a delicious, soothing and healing drink which helps restore the mucous membranes to normal function as well as easing soreness.

Cinnamon, Sassafras, Sarsaparilla, Cloves, Mullein, Licorice root, Aniseed, Fennel and Peppermint may also be added to suit individual tastes and needs. Also eat Garlic fresh, sauteed or in soups in high doses during the acute condition. This will effectively reduce infection in the gastrointestinal tract, and help the formula to do its work within the entire body system.

*Golden Seal root, Burdock root, Lobelia, Mullein, Poke root, Chaparral, Cayenne, Echinacea root(2) and Thyme (0.5)*

## ANTI–INFLAMMATORY FORMULA

Inflammation is the result of congestion of fluids, irritation, injury, infection and abnormal changes in body chemistry. This formula complements the use of the Arthritis and Alkaline formulas as well as formulas which activate the eliminative systems.

Containing White Willow bark, the original, natural source of aspirin, this formula reduces inflammation and pain without providing the side effects of stronger synthetic drugs. The process takes time and must also be coordinated with diet reform and positive changes in living habits. This formula works best when combined with equal parts of Devil's Claw herb.

*White Willow bark, Prickly Ash, Yarrow, Poke root, Elder flowers, Black Cohosh, Nettles, Sarsaparilla and Guiacum*

## ANTI–WEIGHT AND WATER FORMULA

This powerful herbal combination seeks to reduce adipose tissue and eliminate excess water without depleting the system. Once the foundation level of treatment has been achieved and the eliminative channels are working efficiently, this formula will support the restoration to normal body weight by increasing the activity of essential body systems that have become sluggish or overburdened. Once weight and water balance are achieved they can be maintained because of the restoration of normal body function.

Problems such as constant eating, anorexia, bulimia, and mentally and emotionally based cravings and addictions must also be addressed through therapy, counseling and flower essences.

Deep and thorough rejuvenation of the gastrointestinal tract will relieve the physical abnormal and constant hunger caused by non–absorption of nutrients through colon walls which are blocked by impacted faeces. Fatigue and exhaustion also contribute to poor eating habits that cause excess weight and water. Systemic constitutional treatment relieves these conditions by establishing normal function. This formula must be supported by other internal herbal formulas, dietary reform, changes in living habits – the complete holistic health program.

*Burdock root, Bladderwrack (3), Fennel seeds, Echinacea root, Parsley root and Spirulina*

## ARTHRITIS FORMULA

As a complement to systemic treatment, cleansing and diet reform, this formula relieves the discomfort of arthritis and rheumatism. Working to purify the blood, lymph and tissues and reduce inflammation, it helps the system to recover equilibrium of function. The Anti–Inflammatory formula complements the effect of the Arthritis formula.

This formula can also be used as a tea three times a day, or half a cup of the infusion hourly. When discomfort is acute the dosage of capsules may be doubled or tripled.

*Oregon Grape root(2), Parsley root, Sassafras, Prickly Ash bark, Black Cohosh root and Ginger root*

## ASTHMA FORMULA

The treatment of asthma is a challenge to the most qualified and experienced practitioner because it involves cleansing, balancing and activation of the eliminative functions, sensitive counseling for mental and emotional causes, and the introduction of living and dietary habits to lessen mucous formation and support the herbal formula. Treatment for this chronic condition requires the full commitment of the client over about six months. The addition of this formula to systemic treatment steps up the success rate as it encourages the thinning, loosening and expelling of excess mucus from the lungs.

This formula can be taken as a tea (four cups or more per day) depending on need, or in combination with other herbs in capsules or tablets.

It is also useful when used in combination with the Respiratory and Alkaline formulas. Add the Antibiotics Naturally formula if there is evidence of infection, and stop the intake of all mucus forming foods, including sugar, white flour, dairy, coffee, tea and refined, processed foods.

*Slippery Elm, Comfrey root, Marshmallow root, Licorice root and Elecampagne (2)*

## BLOOD PURIFIER FORMULA

Blood purifying herbs help to relieve the blood stream from morbid accumulations which have settled there because of poor dietary and living habits, impaired liver function, and insufficient function of the other eliminative channels, the lymph, bowels, skin and respiratory systems. Whenever the eliminative channels are not functioning properly, toxins accumulate in the blood and tissues and create the climate for infection and disease.

*Echinacea root, Oregon Grape root, Poke root, Red Clover blossoms, Sarsaparilla, Sassafras and Yellow Dock root*

## BODY BUILDING FORMULA

Wherever superior nutrition is needed to provide the raw materials to rebuild damaged or weak bones, muscles and tissue, this formula will provide the means for regeneration. Take internally and apply as poultices directly on affected areas (wounds, damaged vertebrae, broken bones and sprains). If a damaged area does not need to draw nutrients through the blood and lymph, causing congestion, swelling and inflammation, the healing proceeds much more quickly. Because the poultice nutrients are drawn through the skin into the tissues, lymph and circulation of the damaged area, providing nutrients for healing without depleting any other body area or causing excess fluids to be drawn to the damaged areas, inflammation, swelling and pain are reduced and healing progresses more quickly.

*Comfrey root, Comfrey leaves, Irish Moss, Marshmallow root, Mullein, Plantain and White Oak bark*


## BOWEL REJUVENATOR FORMULA

Bowel cleansing and rejuvenation are required by almost every human being on a regular basis. The cleaner the colon, the purer the blood stream and lymph, because the walls of the colon allow the absorption of nutrients into the blood and lymph to be distributed throughout the body. A clean colon gives an uplift physically, mentally and emotionally. One feels lighter, cleaner and clearer, and the brain functions better.

This formula normalizes bowel function, whether the problem is constipation or diarrhea which is an indication of more advanced constipation. A colon that is coated with toxic mucus lining is not able to draw off the fluid containing the nutrients, so the feces become more liquid. When the walls of the colon are clean the liquid can be absorbed in a normal way. If diarrhea is persistent use Mullein tea, high doses of Cinnamon sprinkled on applesauce, or baked potatoes. Symptoms often find their source in the colon, and many chronic diseases owe their early development to the accumulation of bowel toxins. If the causes of ill health are cleared, the way to healing opens. Nutrients become available to the body, and the blood and lymph become cleaner. The burden on the eliminative channels becomes less and one's whole being rejoices. "Cleanliness is next to godliness," the old saying goes.

The aim of this formula is to restore normal bowel function, not to create dependence like most laxatives. Because its ingredients work simultaneously to normalize bowel function, tone colon muscles, restore peristalsis, clean bowel pockets and diverticuli, heal raw or inflamed areas and relax areas of tension, it is an overall formula which will ultimately leave the patient without the need to continue the formula. In some cases bowel cleansing may extend to nine months, but often the colon is cleansed, and normal bowel function is restored, in approximately six months. The iris analysis provides an excellent monitoring of this cleansing process.

The bowels should eliminate three movements a day to ensure that fecal matter is not retained in the bowel for more than twelve hours, and that fermentation and absorption of fecal toxins is minimal.

Because this formula accomplishes a very individual result the dosage must be monitored and adjusted according to response and daily changes. In chronic cases of constipation individuals have taken up to forty–five capsules per day up to three weeks before their body releases its accumulated fecal matter. This initial release can be aided by the use of the Castor oil pack  together with the discriminate use of enemas or colonics.

Caution: Because of its astringent properties Golden Seal should be avoided during pregnancy and nursing, and during regular use should be discontinued after about six weeks. Make the formula without the Golden Seal, add Thyme instead, or use a different bowel formula.

*Cascara Sagrada, Ginger root, Golden Seal (or Thyme), Slippery Elm, Turkey Rhubarb, Wahoo (0.25) and Culver's root (0.25)*

## BOWEL VITALIZER FORMULA

This herbal combination was developed out of a need for a formula which would work as well as Bowel Rejuvenator but not rely on the continued use of Golden Seal, which should not be taken over long periods of time due to its astringent qualities. This formula stimulates bowel elimination through increased liver function. This well–tested formula combines the positive aspects of the Bowel Rejuvenator with a more gentle, less hot, selection of herbs to stimulate natural peristalsis. Adjust dosage according to response. Try out both formula to see which one suits you better, or alternate the Bowel Rejuvenator with the Bowel Vitalizer.

Caution: During pregnancy make up the formula without the Mandrake root.

*Mandrake root, Ginger root, Licorice root, Wild Yam root and Alfalfa*

## BURDOCK

Burdock is a specific herb which is given whenever boils, psoriasis, eczema, itch and other skin diseases present strong symptoms. Its strongly purifying influence also increases urine flow, stimulates the lymphatic system and reduces fatty tissue. Use it together with herbs for the kidneys, liver and bowels to purify the blood.

## CALAMUS

This herb is added to nutrient mixes whenever flatulence, hyperacidity, fermentation, dyspepsia or bloating present strong symptoms. It is very useful for digestive nervous weakness and works efficiently when combined in equal proportions with Gotu Kola.

## CALCIUM FORMULA

A superior intake of calcium is valuable for many conditions including pregnancy, nursing, muscular cramps, hair and nail weakness, and imbalances of body chemistry which lead to weak bones, osteoporosis and calcification of the joints. It is also helpful when babies are teething, because irritability and discomfort are relieved when their bodies have enough calcium to form their teeth without drawing calcium from other areas of their body, causing congestion, pressure on nerves and pain.

*Horsetail (6), Oatstraw (4), Lobelia, Marshmallow root (2), Kelp and Parsley root*

## CAYENNE PEPPER OR CAPSICUM

This stimulant, antiseptic herb has many valuable uses. As a dietary supplement it increases the circulatory power and provides the means to reach sluggish areas. It is also an essential part of any home herbal first aid kit because of its ability to stem the flow of bleeding or hemorrhage. Heart attacks are relieved by high doses of Cayenne because it equalizes the circulation and increases blood flow.

It is worthwhile to learn about the many uses of this excellent herb that is an essential part of many herbal formulas. *Back to Eden* by Jethro Kloss contains a number of pages devoted to its use. Dr. Raymond Christopher found Cayenne so effective that he wrote a book titled *Capsicum*. However, it is important not to overdo the use of Cayenne in formulas or when taken on its own. Extreme use of any herb, however beneficial, will create imbalances and cause reactions.

Caution: Take care when there is sensitivity to hot foods, or if there is liver congestion.

## CHAPARRAL

A North American Indian herb, this desert plant is one of our greatest and strongest herbal purifiers. The rains in the desert release the fragrance of this plant and the air carries its healing aroma and energy. It is good to use Chaparral during purification programs, and whenever there is arthritis or cancer. It accomplishes a deep level of purification and provides healing to both the urinary system and the lower bowel.

However, if this herb is used over a long period of time it will cleanse too drastically and the patient may feel minor distress from an accumulation of mucus in the alimentary tract in the stomach and throat areas. It is best used in strong doses over a short period of time (for example six capsules three times a day for three weeks), and when combined with an ecological nutrient mix that will allow complete elimination of toxins. Chaparral baths are an excellent way of absorbing the nutrient of this powerful purifier directly into the body through the skin.

## CHICKWEED

I once had the opportunity to watch the power of Chickweed at work during an acute crisis. Two days after I had seen a new patient who suffered from severe eczema, I received a telephone call early in the morning. She was hysterical from the pain of itching and heat, crying that when she had these crises before she had to be hospitalized, but she did not want to go to the hospital again. I said "Come right over and we'll see what we can do."

By the time she arrived, I had a Chickweed bath waiting and this sobbing, burning, itching woman, quickly climbed into it. Within seconds the heat and the painful itch were relieved. She soaked for a couple of hours and I sent her away with a large bag of Chickweed. For the next few days she either soaked in a Chickweed bath or was wrapped in cloths soaked in Chickweed infusion. To complement the treatment, she fasted on alkaline juices and herbs. She never had a repeat of this terrible crisis. Over the next few months the condition was cleared by systemic purification and rejuvenation. She eventually changed her stressful job at a mental hospital and created a more relaxed way of life to attain complete healing by eliminating the causes.

Use Chickweed internally and externally to relieve itching and help eliminate the acids which cause burning and itching.

## CHRONIC PURIFIER FORMULA

This formula provides a deep level of blood, tissue and lymph purification in chronic disease, dyscrasia, syphilis and cancer. Use after the eliminative channels are activated and working efficiently.

*Mimosa Gum (2), Echinacea root (3), Blue Flag (3), Comfrey root and Irish Moss*

## CIRCULATION CEREBRAL FORMULA

This formula provides an alternative to the Circulation Systemic formula so that long–term treatment of circulatory disorders do not have to rely on continued use of one formula. Concentrating more on relieving cerebral insufficiency, this formula restores adequate blood flow to the brain areas, relieving tiredness, poor memory, senility and negative mental states.

It is important that it be combined with herbal formulas to discharge morbid accumulations or obstructions in other body areas, organs and systems and to strengthen and support lymph, heart, kidney and liver functions. Every part of the body relies on every other part. When one part of the body is not performing adequately, all the other parts have to adjust and compensate, often to their detriment.

Because poor circulation also affects body temperature and causes the inadequate nourishment of various organs and tissues, it is essential that the circulation be restored if the individual is to regain normal health.

*St. John's Wort, Bayberry, Gingko, Prickly Ash, Cayenne and Sage*

## CIRCULATION SYSTEMIC

The herbs that make up this formula increase the range and power of circulation, especially to deficient areas of the body, the extremities and the capillary circulation. This equalization of the circulation restores normal blood pressure, whether high or low. It is especially important to use this formula to carry herbs to deficient areas if the force of circulation is weak or sluggish. Herbal nutrients travel through the blood and the lymph fluids, so it is essential that all areas of the body receive adequate and regular supplies of blood.

*Bayberry, Cayenne, Ginger root, Golden Seal root and Hawthorn berries*

## COLITIS FORMULA

This formula, together with the Bowel Rejuvenator or Bowel Vitalizer, Nerve and Adrenal formulas, works to unravel the complicated causes of this illness. Counseling is also important along with Bach flower remedies to facilitate changes in mental and emotional attitudes and to ensure that the eliminative channels are all working efficiently.

*Barberry, Golden Seal root, White Oak bark, Myrrh (0. 25), Slippery Elm and Aniseed*

## COLDS AND FLU FORMULA

This formula, together with the Antibiotics Naturally formula, Mustard baths and sweats relieve uncomfortable symptoms, cleanse the system and ensure a quick healing response without the suppression of toxins caused by the use of medical drugs. Supporting the body's acute responses to eliminate accumulated toxins, these herbal aids and associated acute treatments speed recovery and leave the patient stronger and fitter without laying the ground for the development of chronic disease. Hot Ginger, Yarrow or Ephaedra teas are highly recommended for colds or flu. Use the Sore Throat Syrup described in the Antibiotics Naturally formula section.

Drink Elder flowers and Peppermint tea constantly, day and night. Support the elimination with enemas, Mustard baths and steam under quilts to increase perspiration. Use herbal poultices whenever there are lung, throat or glandular complications.

*Elder flowers and Peppermint*

## EAR FORMULA

The combination of the antiseptic qualities of Garlic oil together with the ability of Mullein oil to disperse congested lymph glands around the ear, provides an all–around ear treatment which relieves pain, swelling and infection and also improves hearing quality.

Instructions: drop 4 to 6 drops of each oil into the ear every night and morning for six days. Plug the ear with damp cotton batten. Syringe with equal parts of apple cider vinegar and water on the seventh day – about 10 ml. of each. Repeat this seven–day cycle until the condition is relieved. Support with internal herbal treatment for the immune system and also relieve the cause of the infection in the digestive, circulation and lymphatic systems.

*Mullein and Garlic oils*

## ECHINACEA

This lymphatic herb has a strong and specific power to stimulate lymphatic leukocyte activity. Therefore, its powers for clearing up infection, pus and foul discharges can be used internally and externally wherever tissue decay threatens, or healing repair is slow. It can be added to poultices wherever there is infection. Combine with herbal formula to activate the eliminative channels and strengthen constitutional weakness. It is important to stop the intake of food, clean the bowels with enemas and drink large quantities of herbal purifying teas whenever there are infections.

## ENEMA FORMULA

This formula evolved out of discussions with Margaret Strauss, granddaughter of Dr. Max Gerson, founder of the Gerson Therapy program for cancer and other severe chronic diseases. When I told her about the problems related to adapting their program for strict vegetarian patients, we discussed possible solutions. She clearly felt that if her grandfather had lived longer he would have found vegetarian, herbal substitutions for the coffee enema and the liver and thyroid extracts. She supported the use of my herbal enema formula as an excellent substitute for the coffee enemas.

The added advantage of the herbal enema formula is that superior nutrition is readily available for the direct healing of the walls of the colon, as well as for absorption into the blood and the lymph to be transported throughout the body. After taking this enema one is truly aware of strength and nourishment. The liver is stimulated to dump bile and relieve the system. It also decreases the pain and discomfort of any healing crises.

Instructions: Make a strong decoction by simmering gently one tablespoon Burdock and one tablespoon Yellow Dock root. Turn off the heat. Add one tablespoon Red Clover blossoms and one tablespoon Red Raspberry leaves. Infuse for at least one half hour as it cools. Dilute with distilled water. Inject one quart of the herb mix after the bowel has been cleansed and emptied at least twice with a water enema. Retain five to ten minutes, then expel.

*Red Clover blossoms, Red Raspberry leaves, Burdock root and Yellow dock root*

## EXHAUSTION FORMULA

Although exhaustion has many possible causes – mental, emotional and physical – the treatment of this condition usually requires herbs to aid the digestion and assimilation of nutrients and to strengthen and rebuild the adrenal glands and nervous system.

This formula produces excellent recuperative energy to bring clients back to their normal healthy energy level. The Bach flower remedies, *Olive* and *Hornbeam*, and other flower essences are also a great help. Try a Lobelia bath for deep relaxation. Sleep and rest.

Take Chamomile aromatherapy baths and polarity therapy, acupuncture, cranial sacral, shiatsu and reflexology to release stress and tension. Above all, take a good look at life style. Living in the fast lane and creating burn–out and stress is asking for trouble. Exhaustion is the body calling out for help and change. Its time to break old patterns. Take a vacation, or stay home and sleep all weekend.

You may feel your exhaustion more when you begin taking the herbal nutrients because your true level of energy is revealed. You can no longer push beyond your limits or ignore your body. Discontinue taking any stimulants or caffeine.

*Gentian root (2), Gotu Kola (2), Chondrus Crispus, Cetraria, Alfalfa and Calumba root*

## EYE WASH FORMULA

This eye wash has been successfully used by herbalists for many years for the treatment of cataract, glaucoma, eye weakness and infection. The herbs stimulate circulation to the eyes, relieve congestion, nourish the eyes and cure infection. Although there is sometimes mild stinging when first using the eye wash, this soon passes and the eyes feel bright, refreshed and strengthened. Use one eighth teaspoon of the herb to one half cup water.

Pour boiling water over the herbal powder, steep until it cools, and then strain well through a fine cloth or coffee filter. Using an eye cup, open and close each eye under the infusion for at least one minute. Do this once, twice or three times a day as needed, and continue until the condition is improved. If the eyes are particularly sensitive, dilute the strained infusion further.

*Eyebright and Golden Seal root*

## FEMALE REPRODUCTIVE FORMULA

This herbal combination strengthens, tones, regulates and heals the reproductive organs. Whatever the problem or symptoms, this formula provides the nutrients to support regeneration. It is essential that the eliminative channels be fully cleansed and activated, and that systemic weaknesses are supported if long–term healing is to be achieved. This formula works deeply, relieving cramps, menstrual flooding and pain, and prepares the female reproductive system for healthy childbearing. Combine this formula with the Women's Period Pain formula when cramps and lower backache accompany monthly periods. Combine it with the Menopause or Hormone formulas during the change of life.

*Blue Cohosh, Licorice root, Motherwort, Parsley root, Red Raspberry leaves, Squaw Vine and True Unicorn root*

## FENUGREEK

The highest vegetable source of vitamin D, Fenugreek supports skin rejuvenation programs. Whenever the skin is not eliminating properly, perspiration is insufficient, or the skin is dry and scaly, take six to eight cups of Fenugreek tea a day, one level teaspoon of powder per cup, or simmer the seeds very gently for fifteen minutes and drink throughout the day. The Fenugreek can also be taken in powder or tincture form. This stimulates perspiration and increases gentle elimination. Shower and bathe more often during this treatment, as the skin will eliminates acids and toxins. Take an Epsom salts and cider vinegar bath every other day. After bathing rub the skin with a mixture of almond and wheat germ oil, and scrub the skin twice daily with a natural bristle brush.

## FUNGUS/CANDIDA FORMULA

Although most cases clear during constitutional, eliminative and systemic treatments, when combined with the vaginal ovule and douche, this formula is useful when fungal infections on fingers, feet or elsewhere prove resistant. This formula augments any total approach to clearing the system while helping to relieve irritating symptoms. Use internally and externally as a poultice, bath or douche.

For best results, do not mix herbs or formulas containing seaweeds with this formula as iodine neutralizes the action.

*Thyme, Poke root, Myrrh, Cleavers, Cayenne and Meadowsweet*

## GALL BLADDER FORMULA

This formula completes the gall bladder cleanse given in full detail in *Herbs of Grace*. It should be taken for at least six weeks after the cleanse to reduce inflammation and strengthen and heal the gall bladder.

*Black root, Euonymous, Kava Kava and Marshmallow root (2)*

## GENTIAN

This root is added to eliminative and systemic treatment whenever the absorption of nutrient, digestive weakness or exhaustion are major problems. A strengthening and revitalizing herb, Gentian tones the liver and makes an effective digestive tonic.

## GOTU KOLA

An effective nerve restorative and mental soother, this herb is mixed in equal parts with Calamus when the digestive and nervous systems require combined treatment.

## HAIR STRENGTHENING FORMULA

When hair is weak, brittle or falling out, use this formula to complement systemic treatment. It is essential that the Circulation formula together with purifying herbs also be used to improve the absorption and assimilation of nutrients and their circulation to the head.

Make an herbal tea of Sage, Yarrow and Yellow Dock, using one tablespoon of each herbal powder to one cup of water. Wash the hair while the tea is steeping and then massage it into the hair and scalp. Do not rinse out. Leave it on all day.

In the evening make a mixture of equal parts of Castor oil, wheat germ oil and olive oil, and massage into the head and hair. Steam with hot towels, wrap in a dry towel and leave on all night. Wash the hair well in the morning and then massage in the herb tea again. Leave it on all day. During the day practice inversion postures or slant board exercises. Drink Sage tea, take one or both of the Circulation formula, and take high doses of vitamin E. Continue this treatment for a full seven week cycle and repeat at regular intervals for best results.

*Sage, Yarrow and Yellow Dock root*

## HEART TONIC FORMULA

This normalizing heart formula improves blood pressure, eliminates water retention, strengthens the heart rate, clears arterial deposits, equalizes the force of heart contractions, increases peripheral circulation and beneficially influences the nervous system, providing a wide range of nutrients to balance, strengthen and nourish this hardworking organ. Combine with either or both of the Circulation formulas for best results.

*Hawthorn berries (6), Motherwort (3), Ginseng root (3), Ginger root (2), Comfrey root (2), Lily of the Valley (3), Broom (2), Dandelion leaves(2), Scullcap (2), Lime blossoms (2) and Bugleweed (2)*

## HEAVY METAL PURIFIER FORMULA

After a certain level of eliminative function and systemic balance has been achieved on a six to eight week purification and rejuvenation program, this formula can be given to release a deeper level of cleansing. However, it is essential that all the eliminative channels are working well or the patient will experience headaches, nausea and weakness.

It is important that this formula be combined with the Kidney/Bladder formula, taken on its own between meals with a glass of water or herb tea. Daily Epsom salt baths will increase elimination from the skin. The Heavy Metal formula stimulates the release of toxins which need to be eliminated from the bowels, kidneys, skin, lymph and lungs.

This formula will slowly reduce the shape and size of iris pigmentation markings. Take it over a three week period, rest three weeks, then repeat. The Heavy Metal formula reaches deeply into the tissues to release toxins which have collected in weak areas. If the treatment is guided properly there should be neither discomfort nor weakness as purification progresses.

*Yellow Dock root, Bugleweed, Lobelia, Chaparral and Uva Ursi*

## HORMONE BALANCE FORMULA

The herbs in this formula contain natural hormones offered within complex plant chemistry so that the patients, whether male or female, will be provided with both estrogen and progesterone. The individual body will select what is needed for balance. Use confidently during pregnancy, puberty or menopause, or whenever endocrine functions need tuning.

*Black Cohosh root, Sarsaparilla, Ginseng root, Holy Thistle, Licorice root, False Unicorn root, Squaw Vine and Chasteberry*

## HYDRANGEA

Once one of our British School of iridology graduates was hospitalized with severe kidney pains. After undergoing several days of tests and treatments without improvement and considerable pain, he discharged himself and applied the Hydrangea root treatment. After passing a kidney stone with relative ease, he was cleared of all pain with no recurrence. However, his other eliminative systems were functioning well due to his natural life style. Preparation of the eliminative channels, body organs and systems to a level of active function increases the effectiveness of this treatment. I also advise using the Castor oil pack over the abdomen and the Ginger poultice over the kidneys for at least three days before attempting this treatment. Full instructions are given in the Kidney and Gall Stone Cleanse in the Herbal and Naturopathiy Treatments chapter in *Herbs of Grace*. Use a strong decoction of Hydrangea root to dissolve calcareous kidney stones. Take at least four to six cups daily for seven weeks while following a purification diet and systemic internal herbal treatment guided by an Iridologist.

Individuals have varying tolerances for Hydrangea root, or any specific herb taken in high doses over a length of time. If there are any minor aggravations or signs of toxicity building up, use kineseology or radionics to determine the maximum dose and the length of time to take the Hydrangea root to dissolve the stones. Monitor the dose by being sensitive to body changes and reducing the dose as required. Our program of balanced treatment minimizes such aggravations, but it is always wise to be sensitive, as each person is so individual.

## ILEOCAECAL VALVE FORMULA

This formula regulates over–functioning or under–functioning ileocaecal imbalances. Chiropractors, osteopaths, polarity therapists or applied kineseology practitioners can help to release and adjust this valve. They are also educated about its influence on the digestive system, and the mental and emotional stresses and tensions which aggravate ileocaecal problems. It is essential to treat the nervous system and the adrenals, and take either of the Bowel formula. Abdominal Castor oil packs will also help to relieve symptoms. Lie on the back with the knees up and massage the psoas muscle on either side of the abdomen to release tension.

*Ginger root(0.5), Quassia, Bistort, Bayberry and Angelica root*

## INFECTION FORMULA

Acute infections require high doses of herbs to stimulate the lymphatic system to deal with the invasion. Keep this formula on hand in your first aid kit. For acute infections administer four to six capsules every half hour. Reduce to two capsules for children under twelve years, one capsule for children under seven, and one half capsule for children under two years of age.

This formula is useful for the treatment of colds, flu, fever, abscesses, infected wounds, bronchitis and burns. It is best to have the guidance of a doctor in any serious condition, and certainly if natural medicines are to be used, it is essential that the bowels and stomach are clean and clear. Fast on juices and drink copious amounts of herbal teas.

Whenever there are fevers, clear the bowels with Catnip enemas, soak in a very hot Mustard bath as long as possible, and follow by resting under several blankets in a bed packed with hot water bottles. This encourages a free flow of perspiration, which relieves the system. It is important to stay under the quilts until the body has returned to normal temperature. Drink Yarrow tea during the bath to increase perspiration, and follow with copious amounts of Red

Raspberry, Catnip and Peppermint tea during and after perspiring under the quilts. After the body has cooled, sponge with equal parts of apple cider vinegar and water, and dress in warm cotton clothes. It is beneficial to exercise gently indoors or outdoors, but if there is weakness or sensitivity, return to bed. Clients report that symptoms clear, the fever is reduced quickly and they feel quite well on recovery, without lingering weakness.

*Echinacea root (2), Garlic, Golden Seal root, Lobelia, Mullein and Plantain*

## INTESTINAL INFECTION FORMULA

This formula can be used with bowel cleansing, or to clear intestinal infections from tropical climates. It helps to eliminate harmful microbial parasites and infections in bowel pockets and diverticuli. Although its influence is strong, it is important to have medical tests and consult a doctor or practitioner. Eat large amounts of pumpkin seeds daily (whole or freshly powdered in a coffee grinder) until the condition is cleared. Herbal enemas are also effective.

*Gentian root, Burdock root, Wormwood(2), Sage, Fennel, Mullein, Myrrh, Thyme (2) and Quassia*

## KIDNEY/BLADDER FORMULA

This formula cleanses, heals and balances urine flow, dissolves sediment, tones, and strengthens the function of the entire urinary tract. Kidney problems are not always directly due to kidney weakness. The kidneys also suffer because of the lack of support from other eliminative channels, or because of improper drinking habits. Within the framework of systemic and eliminative treatment, this formula brings the function of the urinary tract to a healthy balanced level.

*Buchu, Clivers, Gravel root, Juniper berries, Marshmallow root, Parsley root and Uva Ursi*

## LADY SLIPPER

One of my favorite herbs, Lady Slipper root is a cerebral sedative that breaks the pattern of stress and strain, gives excellent sleep and relieves emotional sensitivity. It provides a fresh start in the morning, producing a relaxed state which is a relief to any nervous system wound up by work, family or personal crises. It is an excellent aid for jet travel, allowing total relaxation and releasing anxious tensions during the flight, so that travellers arrive fresh and rested. This is a prime remedy for individuals whose illnesses stem from the nervous system. Lady Slipper, now an endangered alpine orchid, is no longer readily available for use individually or in formulas. Valerian is the next best alternative, but for those who can propagate their own supplies of Lady Slipper, their efforts will prove worthwhile.

Dosage: from three to twelve capsules, before sleep or while travelling, depending on the person's age, size, condition and circumstances.

## LADY SLIPPER/VALERIAN

This combination reduces the expense of using pure Lady Slipper and it is also more suitable for those who run on their nerves during the day and are restless and unable to sit down or stop doing things. Divide into three daily doses of two to four capsules per dose. This formula prepares the body to withdraw from tranquilizers or relaxants, and it can also be used before sleep to ensure a good night's rest.

*Lady's Slipper root and Valerian root*

## LIVER/GALL BLADDER FORMULA

The digestive chemical factory needs the full support of liver and gall bladder functions to secrete the alkaline fluids into the duodenum that balance the acid secretions from the pancreas. Together they act on the food that comes from the stomach. This formula begins its work in the stomach and proceeds to influence the digestive process of the liver because it deals with the metabolism of carbohydrates, proteins, fats and the storage and metabolism of vitamins. A healthy liver means clean blood and a good digestion, essential aspects of optimum body function.

The liver also has a strong emotional association with passionate anger, aggression, jealousy and power struggles. It is wise to explore these aggravations and include Bach flower remedies and counseling in holistic treatment.

*Barberry bark (3), Wild Yam root, Cramp bark, Fennel, Catnip, Peppermint, Dandelion root(2), Meadowsweet (2), Wahoo and Black root*

## LYMPHATIC FORMULA

Whenever the lymph system is constitutionally deficient (indicated by a lymphatic rosary in the iris), it is unable to deal with further levels of catarrh created by incorrect diet, high levels of toxins, or invasion by viruses or germs. This formula strengthens and activates the leukocytes, supports the lymph glands, and stimulates balanced elimination. It is important to first consider the level of toxins and the functioning of the other eliminative channels and blood purifying organs, such as the liver and the kidneys, and add appropriate additional formulas as required. Alternate with the Chronic Purifier formula for best results.

*Echinacea root, Lobelia, Mullein, Poke root, Burdock root, Cayenne and Chaparral*

## MENOPAUSE FORMULA

Although every woman and her experience of menopause is unique, this formula offers a background of nourishment, and support for more specific treatment. As well as balancing hormones this formula offers superior nourishment, including natural calcium to help avoid bone loss. It strengthens the kidneys and adrenals, supports the liver and digestive system, relieves hot flashes, eases sore joints and increases energy.

*Alfalfa, Chickweed, Dandelion root, Dong Quai, Fenugreek, Horsetail, Motherwort, Nettles, Red Clover blossoms, Red Raspberry leaves, Violet leaves and Wild Yam root*

## MILK THISTLE

The seeds of this herb can be used to great advantage whenever there is poisoning, chronic skin disease and liver disorders. Add this herb to any program for psoriasis, eczema or liver regeneration. It can also be made into juice from fresh seeds or into powder from dried seeds.

## MUCUS CONGESTION FORMULA

This natural antihistamine relieves irritating sinus and nasal problems associated with colds, flu and hay fever and reduces uncomfortable mucus elimination. Use in combination with the Antibiotics Naturally or the Infection formulas.

**Black Pepper, Aniseed and Ginger root**

## MULLEIN

Diarrhea can be a severe problem during bowel illness and bowel rejuvenation programs. It is essential to use a combination of treatments to reduce the diarrhea as quickly as possible because it is so uncomfortable and debilitating. Mullein tea mixed with hot water or soy milk reduces diarrhea. In stubborn cases also eat a diet of stewed apples with high amounts of cinnamon, baked potatoes and Slippery Elm tea. Astringent enemas or rectal injections of Red Raspberry, Witch Hazel or Bayberry infusions are also useful.

## MULTI-MINERALS/VITAMINS NATURALLY FORMULA

This is a superior balanced herbal alternative to mineral and vitamin supplements! Although our fresh, potent, unprocessed herbal nutrients are richly endowed with vitamins and minerals, this formula contains the full range – a great saving when prices are compared with processed vitamin/mineral supplements. It also contains easily assimilable vegetarian alkaline protein and amino acids. Adjust dose according to need. Two teaspoons provide the equivalent nutrients of a meal and help to take away hunger pangs during healing diets or cleansing fasts.

**Alfalfa, Alkaline formula(4), Anemia formula, Calcium formula(2), Spirulina and Rose hips**

## NERVE REJUVENATOR FORMULA

This formula restores the nervous system and encourages deep rejuvenating sleep. Take two or three capsules two or three time throughout the day. Take six to eight capsules when needed before sleep. It helps rebuild the nervous system after mental or emotional nervous breakdowns.

*Gotu Kola (4), Valerian root (2), Kava Kava, Irish Moss and Lady Slipper root*

## NERVE TONIC FORMULA

Rebuilding the nervous system requires regular intake of nervine herbs, which provide the nutrient for central, autonomic and peripheral nervous systems. Combine this formula with the Calcium, Sweet Sleep or Thyroid formulas if there are problems with hyperactivity or insomnia.

*Catnip, Gotu Kola (2), Lady's Slipper root, Lobelia, Scullcap and Valerian root*

## NERVE VITALIZER FORMULA

This formula strengthens the nervous system during and after trauma, shock, extreme stress, fatigue and accidents.

*Prickly Ash bark (4), Irish Moss and Bayberry bark*

## PAIN RELIEF FORMULA

Whether pain is from acute injuries, headaches, burns, or from chronic diseases like arthritis and rheumatism, this formula will soothe, diminish the discomfort, and encourage sleep. The dose can be adjusted from three times a day with meals to every fifteen minutes, one–half hour, or every hour as needed. It works best in combination with professionally guided treatment to relieve the cause of the pain. Dosage: one to four capsules as needed.

*White Willow bark, Jamaican Dogwood, Valerian root and Cramp bark*

## PANCREAS FORMULA

The herbs in this formula offer natural insulin that helps to lower blood sugar levels and strengthen and feed this gland. Use this formula as part of a holistic systemic program. Hypoglycemia will also be relieved by this formula, especially if several cups of Licorice tea are drunk throughout the day. Eat vegetarian, alkaline, fresh organic food and fresh juices.

*Elecampagne (2), Golden Seal root, Uva Ursi, Wahoo (2), Licorice root, Mullein, Nettles, Allspice and Juniper berries*

## PROLAPSE FORMULA

There are many factors which contribute to a prolapsed colon condition. The case history and iridology reading will help to determine whether it is related to weak connective tissue, pressure from other organs, bowel toxins or nutritional deficiency. Internal herbal treatment can be supported by specific feeding of the pelvic area by the use of ovules and douches.

*Black Cohosh, Witch Hazel, White Oak bark (2), Lobelia, Yellow Dock and Marshmallow root*

## PSYLLIUM

Soak one teaspoon of Psyllium seeds in one–half cup of warm water. Add juice to improve the taste if you wish. This mucilaginous mixture sweeps the bowel walls clean and provides bulk to ease constipation. Take concurrently with either of the Bowel formulas, during a bowel cleanse treatment, but do not use on a regular long–term basis.

## RESPIRATORY FORMULA

This formula supports the respiratory system when it is actively eliminating, infected or chronically weak from conditions like asthma and bronchitis. It works best when it is combined with the Asthma formula, as well as systemic treatment for activating and cleansing the eliminative channels and purifying and regenerating the body systems and organs.

*Comfrey root, Elecampagne, Elder flowers, Mullein (2), Licorice root and Lobelia*

## SKIN PROBLEMS FORMULA

Chronic skin problems are deep–seated and involve all the blood purifying organs, the eliminative channels and the defense systems of the skin itself. This deeply purifying formula works well in combination with systemic treatment to eliminate morbid conditions from the blood that cause the skin to suffer the consequences. It is also essential to improve the diet. Add the following to the program: the Bowel Rejuvenator, Liver/Gall Bladder, and Kidney/Bladder formulas, and Milk Thistle seeds.

*Blue Flag, Burdock root, Burdock seeds, Cayenne, Echinacea root, Poke root and Red Clover blossoms*

## SLIPPERY ELM

Whenever a sensitive digestive system reacts against food or herbs, Slippery Elm forms the perfect carrier to reduce discomfort. Make a warm drink of one teaspoon Slippery Elm powder with one cup of warm soy milk or water, and add honey, maple syrup, Carob or Cinnamon as desired to improve the taste. Mix and drink immediately, before it becomes too thick. As well as soothing and protecting the intestinal wall and easing digestion, this herbal nutrient is a highly nutritious food which contains abundant calcium.

This mucilaginous herb is also used with poultices and the vaginal ovule because it helps to hold the herbal powders together.

## SMOKING FORMULA

This formula reduces the need for nicotine, alters taste cravings so that the desire for smoking is reduced and relieves pain in the respiratory system. I have known many patients who have completely stopped smoking after using this mix. Roll into a handmade herbal 'cigarette' and smoke!

The smoking mix is also excellent for relieving respiratory pain in chronic lung diseases. The Lobelia relaxes the chest and disperses congestion, while the Mullein soothes, heals and comforts. Lobelia poultices are an excellent complement to this treatment.

*Coltsfoot, Mullein, Yerba Santa and Lobelia*

## SPIRULINA

This nutritious algae contains almost every mineral and vitamin required in our diet, including a high amount of B vitamins and assimilable alkaline protein. Whenever there is weakness, exhaustion, strong cravings or hunger, this food helps to balance digestion. It is an excellent supplement to use during fasts, juice cleanses and purifying diets.

## STOMACH ACID/ALKALINE BALANCING FORMULA

Imbalances of body chemistry often begin in the stomach. Whether the stomach is too acid or too alkaline this formula will provide the wide range of nutrients necessary to normalize the stomach environment. It is also useful to add this formula wherever the digestion is sensitive because it helps soothe and heal the stomach and ease other herbs into the system.

*Dandelion root, Slippery Elm, Calamus, Meadowsweet, Irish Moss and Iceland Moss*

## SWEET SLEEP FORMULA

Restful sleep depends to a large extent on the ability of our parasympathetic nervous system to relax and release us from the stress and strain of daily activities. These herbs mildly sedate the nervous system and encourage a sweet restful sleep that leaves one rested, yet alert in the morning. During times of stress or intense activity, this formula can also be taken with food at regular intervals during the day.

*Passion flowers, Lady Slipper root, Valerian root, Scullcap, Hops, Broom and Lime tree flowers*

## Swollen Glands Formula

Use this formula internally, and as a fomentation to relieve congestion and reduce swelling and discomfort. Use with the Lymphatic and Antibiotics Naturally formulas for best results. Leave the fomentation on all night and day if necessary, six days a week.

*Lobelia, Mullein (2), Parsley root or leaves and Plantain*

## Tableting Formula

Use with tableting rollers and cutters, or for hand–rolled tablets. This formula will reduce sticking and finish the tablets with a tasty nutritive powder. Sprinkle carob on the tablets to further improve the taste.

*Alkaline formula (2), Slippery Elm and Cinnamon or Carob*

## Thyroid Balancing Formula

Whether the thyroid is underactive or overactive, the body, mind and emotions become disturbed if this master gland does not receive the nutrients required for balanced activity. Use this formula together with the Adrenal, Sweet Sleep, or Nerve formulas for an overactive thyroid, or with the Exhaustion and Multi–Mineral formulas if the thyroid is underactive.

*Parsley leaves, Kelp (2), Irish Moss, Iceland Moss, Nettles, Bladderwrack
and Bugleweed*

## Vaginal Ovule Formula

The vaginal ovule is an internal poultice which is used to transform the environment of the vagina, to offer superior healing nutrition and to draw out toxic poisons from the tissues, blood and lymph. Although the deeper cause may be inherited, or the result of mental, emotional and living influences combined with systemic toxicity, much can be gained by using the ovule locally to relieve chronic reproductive conditions, discharges, irritation, itching and sores. The ovule also positively influences deeper conditions such as cysts, tumors, inflammation, sores and cervical dysplasia, providing nutrients for healing exactly where they are needed.

The herbs are absorbed into the mucus membranes and spread via the capillary circulation and lymph into the pelvis. When the ovule is supported with herbal nutrients taken internally, the influences meet, contributing to total healing. Visualize the pelvis as an environment where everything touches everything else, where either toxins or healing can spread out from the bowels through the circulation of lymph and blood. Emotional and muscular tensions in the solar plexus also inhibit peristalsis. If healing is to take place the pelvis must be cleansed and restored to harmonious function within the total ecology of the whole person. Refer to the instructions on page xxxii at the end of this appendix.

*Squaw Vine, Echinacea root, Comfrey root, Marshmallow root, Chickweed
and Golden Seal root*

## WILD YAM

Whenever flatulence, gas, wind, spasms, colic or stomach discomfort contribute strong symptoms, this root is added to the herbal nutrient mix. It is also excellent for uterine cramps. It can be taken together with the Women's Period Pain formula throughout pregnancy both as a tonic and to prevent miscarriage. This herb is also a natural source of progesterone precursors and has applications for women's reproductive and hormonal conditions and menopause.

## WOMEN'S PERIOD PAIN FORMULA

If cramps and pain disturb your menstrual cycle, use this formula just before your period is due and during any discomfort. Because the effect is accumulative, the need for it should lessen from month to month, especially if the causes are being relieved by systemic purification and rejuvenation. Chamomile tea will also help relieve cramps when it is taken immediately.

*Blue Cohosh, Cramp bark (2), Lemon Balm, Ginger root, Turmeric and Valerian root*

## YELLOW DOCK

Yellow Dock root is used for the douche which supports the Vaginal Ovule treatment. Its high iron content attracts oxygen, increases cellular metabolism and restores health to the mucus membrane. It is also part of the Anemia formula which is taken throughout pregnancy. An herbal decoction made from the root or tea made from powdered root are excellent ways to take iron in an easily assimilable form. A valuable blood–purifying herb and a lymphatic stimulant, Yellow Dock contributes a positive influence whenever it is used.

## HERBAL DECOCTIONS

Decoctions are strong herbal brews that bring out the virtues from whole or cut roots, barks and berries. When they are powdered they can be infused or simmered gently for a short time and then left to steep. Decoctions are used for drinks, baths, enemas, poultices and fomentations.

If you wish to make a decoction of cut or whole berries, roots or barks and the plant material is not powdered, simmer the herb very, very gently over a very low flame so that the virtue of the herb or herbs will be released without destroying the potency or value. Use only glass or stainless steel containers. Small seeds like Fenugreek need about twenty minutes, and roots which are very hard may take about thirty to forty–five minutes.

Decoction proportions are approximately thirty grams, or one ounce of herb, per one pint of water, or one–half ounce per cup. Start out with two pints so that one pint will boil off during the simmering.

## HERBAL TEAS, TISANES OR INFUSIONS

Herbal teas are used for many purposes; delightful drinks, enemas, baths, poultices, and as medicinal support during acute crises or chronic conditions. They can be made from powders, leaves, roots and barks or even from tinctures or aromatherapy oils. They can be individual herbs, mixtures of two or more herbs, or formulas made up of numerous herbs. The best approach is to start simple, try a few herbs, get to know them, and then expand the repertoire. It is best to try recipes and commercial blends until we find our way and learn to enjoy the creative art of natural herbal beverage blending.

Proportions vary according to taste and depend upon the part of the plant used, its purpose, freshness and potency. The general rule is to use one teaspoon of herb per cup of tea. Many prefer half that amount of herb for enjoyment and double that when there is a medicinal need. If you are using the herbal teas for enemas, poultices, baths or fomentations, use a higher dose of herbs per cup of liquid, from one to two teaspoons per cup of liquid.

Pour boiling water over the herbs. Use a glass or stainless steel tea pot so that chemical reactions will not take place within the container. Porous metals such as aluminum are unsuitable for use with herbs. Steep longer than for ordinary tea, at least twelve minutes. Pour off the beverage through a strainer. Glass tea pots make elegant containers that show off the beauty and color of the herbs. Add flowers like hibiscus, chrysanthemum, violets or rose petals for beauty and fragrant taste.

Leave the herbs in the container and add fresh amounts of boiling water, then add more herbs as required during the day. Clean out the pot at the end of the day and start fresh the next morning. Honey or maple syrup is pleasant. If you are using barks or roots and they are not ground into a powder, make a decoction, strain and add into the tea. Don't mix them during the preparation.

If you are having a party and want to serve a delightful herbal juice punch, try my favorite recipe: apple juice, red grape juice, orange and lemon juice mixed with Hibiscus, Lemon Grass, Peppermint, Ginger and Rose Hips. Add a dash of Cinnamon and Allspice. Float a few orange and lemon rings, mull to a moderate, warm temperature, or serve iced. Your guests will appreciate this delicious and satisfying drink.

# Herbal Tea Formulas

DIGESTEA – This delightful tea improves the digestive chemistry, balances the acid/alkaline secretions in the stomach, improves digestion and increases the assimilation of nutrients. Take a cup one quarter hour before, or half an hour after, eating or anytime throughout the day.

*Meadowsweet, Wood Betony, Peppermint, Hibiscus, Lemon Grass, Rose Hips and Fennel*

SERENITEA – If you would like to relax before sleep, try one or two cups of this tea before retiring. Because it is a strong but pleasant tasting tea, milk and honey improves the flavor. This is a useful tea to have on hand to weather stress, crises or emotional upsets.

*Catnip, Vervain, Mistletoe, Peppermint, Wood Betony (3), Valerian (0.5),*
*Scullcap (0.5) and Hops (0.5)*

WATERBALANCE – This mildly diuretic tea beneficially influences the entire urinary tract and helps regulate the elimination of water. Acute cystitis can be helped by drinking a cup every half an hour until the symptoms are relieved.

*Couchgrass, Parsley Leaves, Clivers, Buchu, Uva Ursi and Chickweed*

# Individual Herbal Teas

*Chickweed* – Neutralizes and eliminates acidity.

*Ginger* – Fresh Ginger increases body heat and improves digestion.

*Licorice* – A gentle aperient for children and adults that also stabilizes blood sugar; take six cups a day for hypoglycemic conditions.

*Mullein* – Slows diarrhea and balances bowel function.

*Oat Straw* – A high source of silica and calcium, add it to teas and use in water cure full baths and footbaths.

*Red Clover* – An excellent blood purifier that combines well with Red Raspberry during purification programs.

*Red Raspberry* – The high iron content attracts oxygen and increases metabolic activity, overcoming sluggishness; excellent for pregnant women; add to teas during pregnancy and for strength during and after menstrual periods.

*Rose Hips* – Add to tea blends to provide vitamin C during colds and infections.

*Sage* – This ancient Chinese longevity tea stimulates cerebral circulation and increases brain activity and memory.

## OILS AND OINTMENTS

*Balm of Gilead Ointment* – Soothes and heals eczema, psoriasis, sores, cracked skin and open wounds.

*Chickweed Ointment* – Relieves heat, itching and rashes.

*Comfrey Ointment* – Aids cell growth, and the repair of cuts, wounds and fractures; provides regenerative nutrients directly where it is needed.

*Garlic Oil* – Useful for warts, pimples and infected wounds; apply directly on areas two to three times per day; combine with Mullein oil for ear infections.

*Mullein Oil* – Two to three drops in the ear relieve earache, suppuration and inflammation of the ear, especially when combined with Garlic oil. It can also be applied externally on sprains, bruises, sores, swollen glands, aching joints and skin diseases.

## BATHS, FOOTBATHS AND HAND BATHS

During my studies and purifications at *Rainbow Island* and *Healing Waters* healing centers, we bathed regularly in Chaparral herbal baths, absorbing the purifying herb directly through our skin. Lobelia baths produce deep relaxation during crises, trauma or exhaustion. Chickweed baths relieve itching and skin discomfort. Hand and foot baths draw the nutrients immediately into the capilliary circulation and then quickly into the blood stream. Make herbal baths an important part of home therapeutics.

## HERBAL TINCTURES

*ANTISPASMODIC* – Useful for shocks, cramps, spasms, hysteria, asthma and heart attacks.

*Lobelia, Scullcap, Black Cohosh, Cayenne, Gum Myrrh, Catnip and Cramp Bark*

*DIGESTIVE* – Relieves colic, wind and discomfort in the stomach. Excellent for children.

*Catnip and Fennel*

*NERVINE NUTRIENT* – Feeds and calms the nervous system and reduces hyperactivity. Rub on the back of the neck to influence the medulla regulatory center and calm breathing and basic body functions.

*Black Cohosh, Lady's Slipper, Scullcap, Lobelia and Blue Vervain*

*NERVINE RELAXANT* – Calms the nervous system when sleep or digestion are disturbed.

*Wild Lettuce and Valerian*

## INDIVIDUAL HERBAL TINCTURES

*Echinacea* – Assists the lymphatic defense system during acute infections, colds, flu.

*Euphrasia* – An excellent eye wash to brighten and strengthen the eyes.

*Elder flower* – The highest herbal source of potassium, Elderflower complements treatment for excess acidity, fibroids and nutritional imbalance; helps to maintain a youthful and supple skin.

*Lobelia* – By prescription only, for use as an internal emetic when combined with Peppermint tea (do not attempt an emetic without professional advice), and to relieve asthma by rubbing over congested areas to relieve pain, spasms and swelling; use as a poultice over the lung area to relieve congestion, inflammation, pain and coughing.

*Myrrh* – Rub into gums after brushing the teeth or use a dropper in dental cleaning equipment solutions; good for bleeding gums, pyorrhea, sores, pimples and herpes.

*Saw Palmetto* – A specific for the mammary glands, it complements treatment for breast lumps and swollen breasts. Take internally and rub on the breasts.

*Wild Yam* – Relieves digestive flatulence, bloating, colic and cramps; high in progesterone; useful to relieve hot flashes, prevent osteoporosis and balance hormones during menopause.

## TINCTURE DOSAGE

Drop the tincture dose in a glass and pour boiling water over it. Steep at least five minutes so that the alcohol can be evaporated before drinking. Swish it around in the mouth, allowing the taste buds to benefit from the flavor as it is mixed with saliva, then swallow. Tinctures are administered according to age, three to four times per day as required or more often in acute conditions. Size, weight and sensitivity are also considerations.

*The full adult dose is:*

Use six, twelve or eighteen drops in water, three, six or nine times daily as required.

*Acute Conditions:*

Dosage can be increased to every five, ten or fifteen minutes minutes, half hour, hour, and so on, depending on the need, symptoms and response. Seek professional guidance.

# CASTOR OIL PACKS

Castor oil packs assist in cleansing and clearing the bowels. The absorption of the Castor oil through skin pores into the lymph system softens, relaxes and nourishes the bowels, as well as balancing the sympathetic and parasympathetic nervous systems, when it is absorbed into the lacteals in the small intestine. It also disperses congestion, relieves tension and helps to release any blockages or bowel pockets.

Dr. Raymond Christopher states in his book *School of Natural Healing*: "Castor oil helps to get rid of hardened mucus in the body, which may appear as cysts, tumors or polyps." Many patients resist this treatment because they fear it will be messy. When they finally do it and are rewarded by the results, they always wish they had done it earlier. Follow these instructions:

1. To prevent stains, place a towel over a piece of plastic to protect the chair or the bed.
2. Cover a cookie tin, or similar flat surface, with a plastic baggie.
3. Place a white cotton cloth or dish towel (no dyed colors) over the baggie.
4. Pour warmed Castor oil over the cloth, soaking it thoroughly without making it too wet. Fold the cloth to spread the oil evenly and then unfold it fully onto the plastic which has been placed on the cookie tin.
5. Cover the oil–soaked cloth with a second water moistened cotton cloth.
6. Cover these two layers of cloth with another baggie or piece of plastic. Lift them all off the bottom plastic bag, turn and place the Castor oil cloth directly on the skin. The moist cotton cloth remains in the middle with a baggie on top, so the final layer of thick towel will not be stained by the oil. Sometimes the oil runs out the side as the heat increases, so make sure the surface you are sitting or lying on is well protected as suggested above. The layers from the skin out are: oil–soaked cloth, damp cloth, plastic baggie and then the towel.
7. Place the heating pad over all of this. Hot water bottles can also be used but they are not so convenient because they are heavy, cool quickly and need refilling during the treatment. Don't fill hot water bottles too full, or they will feel heavy and uncomfortable, and will not lie flat on the abdomen.
8. Cover everything with another thick towel or blanket which wraps around the body to hold everything in place and to help retain the heat.
9. Enjoy this soothing and relaxing pack for one–and–one–half hours, three days in a row. Each day place the two layers of cotton and the top layer of plastic back on the protective layer of plastic on the cookie tin, then roll it up and put it away. Put new Castor oil on the cloth each time you apply it, taking care not to make it too oily.
10. For the next three days, massage the entire abdominal area with olive oil.
11. Wash the cloths and leave them in the sun and air to purify for at least one day.
12. Rest on the seventh day. Repeat the entire procedure again.

Enjoy the Castor oil pack by reading, writing, resting, meditating, watching television or videos, or sleeping while the pack is on. The relaxation of the solar plexus is very soothing, and especially valuable to release the kind of constipation caused by muscular tension. Make a strong effort to overcome any resistance to doing the Castor oil pack, and include it in any home care program.

Buy solid coconut oil from a health food store or deli. Soften it over low heat. Add in one drop of Tea Tree oil. Combine a week's supply of the vaginal ovule formula powder with an equal amount of Slippery Elm powder. Mix well by shaking both together in a plastic bag. Mix the oil with the powder until you obtain a doughy paste. Place the mixture on a sandwich baggie and roll into a long tube. The baggie keeps your hands clean and gives a smooth finish to the ovule. Cut the tube into one inch lengths. Wrap with the baggie. Keep them in the refrigerator.

Ovules stay relatively solid inside the vagina. Remove the ovule with a finger or the douches. Plug the opening of the vagina with cotton wool, a homemade tampon of natural sea sponge, or an end cut from a tampon. Press on the plug so that it won't come out during bowel movements.

Wear black underpants during this treatment, so they are not ruined by stains. Some women may also need to wear a mini–pad.

Although we recommend abstaining from sexual intercourse during the vaginal treatment, if partners cannot wait to make love, do so after removing the ovule and douching with Yellow Dock. Douche again after making love, then continue the program.

*Monday a.m.*

Insert one to three one–inch ovules, depending on the size of the vagina. Leave in all day. Hold in place with a sponge or cut tampon. Replace it if it comes out. Insert a fresh ovule and leave it in all night. Insert a new ovule on Tuesday morning after moving the bowels.

*Tuesday p.m.*

Douche the vagina with one cup of well strained Yellow Dock or Burdock infusion. Lie in the bath to keep warm and relaxed. Lift the pelvis up. Retain the fluid inside the vagina at least five minutes so that it can be absorbed into the mucus membranes, tissues, blood and lymph. Visualize that the ovules are spreading their positive influence into the pelvis. Add Thyme tea or Tea Tree oil if there are Candida or thrush problems. Insert another ovule into the vagina. Leave in overnight until Wednesday morning.

*Wednesday, Thursday and Friday*

Repeat the Monday and Tuesday procedures until Saturday.

*Saturday p.m.*

Remove the ovule, douche, but do not insert another ovule until Monday morning, when the entire procedure is repeated for up to a period of seven weeks, then have a break. Many patients report that not much happens until the third or fourth week. Discharges, odors and other reactions are normal as toxins and mucus are released. Support the treatment with internal herbs and a purification diet.

Continue the ovule treatment throughout the monthly menstrual cycle. When the flow is heavy, count the days of strong flow and resume the same weekly schedule when the flow is light. You also can replace the ovule more often, or use it just at night.

# Index

# SCHOOL OF NATURAL MEDICINE STUDY OPPORTUNITIES

## HOME STUDY

Correspondence courses in Iridology, Herbal Medicine and Naturopathy and a combined Natural Physician course are available worldwide from the School of Natural Medicine. Contact us for brochure, newsletters, and the latest prices and class schedules.

TEL: (888) 593–6173   FAX: (888) 593–6733
email: snm@purehealth.com   website: www.purehealth.com

## SUMMER SCHOOLS

A summer program is held every August presenting the entire system of natural medicine, including Iridology, Naturopathy and Herbology, with special workshops in Elemental Energetics, an in–depth study of the elements of life that make up our body and our world, and clinical training. Send for the brochure for full details, dates and fees. The classes also include herbal apprentice training with expert wilderness, wildcrafting and herbal teachers, and hands–on training in the Herbs of Grace pharmacy and dispensary.

## SEMINARS

Advanced seminars in clinical training, mystic yoga and dance, transformational movement, and living foods teacher training are held yearly. Check out the website for school programs and international seminars .

## TRANSFORMATIONAL JOURNEYS:

The school organizes trips, transformational healing, and educational journeys to India, Puerto Rico, Greece, and Mexico. Some of these journeys also fulfill requirements for the Naturopathy diploma (ND).

## CLINIC:

The school offers consultations to guide clients to become independently healthy.

## HERBS OF GRACE:

The school pharmacy dispensary offers quality herbal formulae to students and clients.

*Companion volume...*

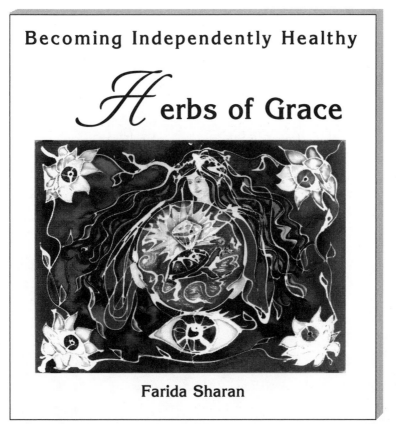

# Becoming Independently Healthy

# *H*erbs of Grace

### Farida Sharan

*4 color laminate cover • Size 7 5/8 x 9 1/8 • 224 pages • Index • Illustrations • ISBN 1–57093–003–1 • LCCN 94–76389*

**POSTAGE & PAYMENT INFORMATION**
*Herbs of Grace - Becoming Independently Healthy $23.95*
Order from www.purehealth.com or amazon.com

NAME ................................................................................................ TEL. NO. ...............................................

ADDRESS ...........................................................................................................................................................

....................................................................................... CITY......................................................................

STATE ....................................................................... ZIP CODE ............................... .COUNTRY ...............................

VISA/MASTERCARD NUMBER ........................................................................ EXPIRATION DATE ...........................

NUMBER OF BOOKS ........... X  $23.95 EACH                    $ .................

NUMBER OF BOOKS ........... X CORRECT POSTAGE/ BOOK $ ............... $ ................    **TOTAL  $ .................**

SIGNATURE ...................................................................................... DATE ................................

**Wisdome Press, a division of School of Natural Medicine**
**TEL: (888) 593–6173  *  FAX: (888) 593–6733**

# MENOPAUSE ORDER FORM

## HERBAL FORMULAS RECOMMENDED DURING MENOPAUSE

| | |
|---|---|
| Adrenal | $_____ |
| Body Building | $_____ |
| Bowel Rejuvenator | $_____ |
| Calcium | $_____ |
| Endometriosis Complex | $_____ |
| Exhaustion | $_____ |
| Heart | $_____ |
| Hormone Balancing | $_____ |
| Kidney/Bladder | $_____ |
| Liver/Gall Bladder | $_____ |
| Lymphatic | $_____ |
| Menopause | $_____ |
| Nerve Rejuvenator | $_____ |
| Vege capsules – 500 (size 00) | $_____ |
| Capsuling machine | $_____ |
| Shipping & Handling | $_____ |
| Books (listed below) | $_____ |
| TOTAL | $_____ |

*Creative Menopause – Illuminating Women's Health & Spirituality*  $17.95

*Flower Child*  $18.95

*Herbs of Grace – Becoming Independently Healthy*  $23.95

*Iridology – A Complete Guide*  $50.00

PLEASE CONTACT US FOR LATEST PRICES OF HERBS & SHIPPING CHARGES.

NAME_____

ADDRESS_____

_____ZIP CODE_____COUNTRY_____

TELEPHONE_____ FAX_____

VISA/MASTERCHARGE #_____EXPIRATION DATE_____

NAME ON CARD_____ SIGNATURE_____

**Herbs of Grace, a division of School of Natural Medicine**
**TEL: (888) 593–6173  *  FAX: (888) 593–6733**
**email: snm@purehealth.com  website: www.purehealth.com**

# HERBS OF GRACE HERB ORDER FORM

The School of Natural Medicine's herbal pharmacy, Herbs of Grace, offers safe, non–toxic, non–habit forming herbal nutrient formulas created by Dr. Farida Sharan. The wildcrafted, organic, fresh ground herbal powders are blended to order, to the highest professional standard. Powders provide the purest, most easily assimilable herbal food without the addition of alcohol or the chemical changes of the extraction process. All formulas have been tried and tested by hundreds of our graduates and professionals. Complete details on all the formulas, contents and recommended use, together with information on diets and home naturopathic treatments are provided in *Herbs of Grace – Becoming Independently Healthy*, which may be requested with the herb order. Capsules and capsuling machines may also be ordered.

| # | Powders or capsules per ounce | $ | $ Total | # | Powders or capsules per ounce | $ | $ Total |
|---|---|---|---|---|---|---|---|
| ___ | Adrenal | | ___ | ___ | Menopause | | ___ |
| ___ | Alkaline | | ___ | ___ | Multi-Mineral/Vitamins | | ___ |
| ___ | Allergy | | ___ | ___ | Nerve Rejuvenator | | ___ |
| ___ | Anemia | | ___ | ___ | Nerve Tonic | | ___ |
| ___ | Antibiotic | | ___ | ___ | Nerve Vitalizer | | ___ |
| ___ | Anti–Weight | | ___ | ___ | Pancreas Sugar Balance | | ___ |
| ___ | Anti–Inflammatory | | ___ | ___ | Prolapse | | ___ |
| ___ | Arthritis | | ___ | ___ | Prostate | | ___ |
| ___ | Asthma | | ___ | ___ | Respiratory | | ___ |
| ___ | Bloood Purification | | ___ | ___ | Skin Clear | | ___ |
| ___ | Body Building | | ___ | ___ | Stomach Acid/Alkaline Balance | | ___ |
| ___ | Bowel Rejuvenator | | ___ | ___ | Sweet Sleep | | ___ |
| ___ | Bowel Activator | | ___ | ___ | Thyroid | | ___ |
| ___ | Calcium | | ___ | ___ | Vaginal Ovule +Y.D. + S.Elm | | ___ |
| ___ | Chronic Purifier | | ___ | ___ | Women's Period Pain | | ___ |
| ___ | Circulation Systemic | | ___ | ___ | Capsuling Machine | | ___ |
| ___ | Circulation Cerebral | | ___ | ___ | *Herbs of Grace* book | | ___ |
| ___ | Colitis | | ___ | ___ | *Creative Menopause* book | | ___ |
| ___ | Enema Mix | | ___ | ___ | *Flower Child* book | | ___ |
| ___ | Exhaustion | | ___ | ___ | 500 Vegetarian Capsules | | ___ |
| ___ | Female Reproductive | | ___ | ___ | School Brochure | | ___ |
| ___ | Fungal Infection | | ___ | | | | |
| ___ | Heart | | ___ | | TOTAL | | ___ |
| ___ | Heavy Metal Purifier | | ___ | | POSTAGE | | ___ |
| ___ | Hormone Balance | | ___ | | GRAND TOTAL | | ___ |
| ___ | Ileo-Caecal Valve | | ___ | | | | |
| ___ | Intestinal Infection | | ___ | | | | |
| ___ | Kidney/Bladder | | ___ | LET US KNOW WHETHER YOU WANT THE HERBS: | | | |
| ___ | Liver/Gall Bladder | | ___ | packaged separately OR blended together; | | | |
| ___ | Lymphatic | | ___ | as powders OR in vege caps | | | |

## POSTAGE & PAYMENT INFORMATION
### Contact us for latest prices and shipping charges

DATE ........................................................... AMOUNT IN FULL ...........................................

NAME ............................................................................ TEL. NO. ...........................................

ADDRESS ...............................................................................................................................

.......................................... ZIP CODE ............................ COUNTRY ...................................

VISA/MASTERCARD NUMBER ................................................... EXPIRATION DATE ...................

SIGNATURE ............................................................................................................................

**TEL: (888) 593-6173  FAX: (888) 593-6733**
**website: www.purehealth.com   email: snm@purehealth.com**

# Educational Programs

**HOME STUDY COURSES** – includes the books mentioned below

Iridology and the Foundation of Natural Medicine (MIr)

Herbal Medicine (MH)

Naturopathy (ND)

Natural Physician – all 3 home courses and all the books and slides

**SUMMER SCHOOL** – Elements of Life, Iridology, Naturopathy, Herbal Medicine & Clinical Training

**COMPLETE PACKAGE** – 3 Home Study Courses & Summer School

**SEMINARS & ADVANCED TRAINING** – Offered throughout the year

**HEALING JOURNEYS** – Offered throughout the year

**MYSTIC YOGA & DANCE** – Ongoing classes throughout the year

CONTACT US FOR CURRENT COURSE PRICES

# Books & Slides

| | |
|---|---|
| Iridology – *A Complete Guide* | $55.00 |
| Herbs of Grace – *Becoming Independently Healthy* | $23.95 |
| Iridology Coloring Book – Safi & Sharan, learn by coloring beautiful iris drawings | $33.00 |
| Dictionary of Iridology – Safi's visual reference of Sharan's Iridology course | $33.00 |
| Creative Menopause – *Illuminating Women's Health & Spirituality* | $17.95 |
| Flower Child – Spiritual Memoir of healing transformation in the 60's | $18.95 |
| Slide Set – 15 color 35 mm slides with matching iris drawings to color, and case histories | $45.00 |

CONTACT US FOR CURRENT SHIPPING & HANDLING CHARGES

VISA/MASTERCHARGE #...........................................................EXPIRATION DATE........................

NAME.......................................................................................DATE .................................

ADDRESS....................................................................................................................

.............................Zip code.....................Country.....................................Tel:................................

SIGNATURE.........................................................TOTAL PAYMENT $...........................

**SCHOOL OF NATURAL MEDICINE**
TEL: (888) 593–6173 * FAX: (888) 593–6733
email: snm@purehealth.com   website: www.purehealth.com